MW00709531

Healing Planet Earth

Macrobiotics and the New Ecology

By Edward Esko
Foreword by Alex Jack

One Peaceful World Press
Becket, Massachusetts

*For Eric, Balinda, Mark, Daniel, Thomas, Julia, Matthew, Amanda,
Elizabeth, Cristofer, Peter, Senin, and Future Generations*

For further information on mail-order sales, wholesale or retail dis-
counts, distribution, translations, and foreign rights, please contact
the publisher:

One Peaceful World Press
P.O. Box 10
Leland Road
Becket, MA 01223
U.S.A.

Telephone (413) 623-2322
Fax (413) 623-8827

First Edition: May 1996
10 9 8 7 6 5 4 3 2 1

ISBN 1–882984–20-X
Printed in U.S.A.

Contents

4

Foreword

There are many dimensions to the global environmental crisis: destruction of the rain forests; thinning of the ozone layer; contamination of the soil with pesticides and chemical fertilizers; pollution of oceans, lakes, and streams; acid rain; desertification and drought; decline of biodiversity and the extinction of many plants and animals; changing weather patterns and unusual seasonal changes; the spread of infectious disease; and global warming.

While there are many approaches to these problems, the most fundamental solution is a change in the modern way of eating to a diet high in whole cereal grains and other plant quality foods and low in animal products and other highly refined, energy-intensive foods. Around the world, ecologists, environmentalists, and others concerned with these issues are shifting to a macrobiotic, semi-macrobiotic, or more vegetarian diet as the single most practical step one can take to help restore planetary, as well as personal, health.

In Healing Planet Earth, Edward Esko explains how the modern food industry and modern agriculture are directly linked to environmental destruction and how a naturally balanced diet is an essential aspect of both an ecologically-aware and a health-conscious lifestyle.

The first edition of *Healing Planet Earth* was published in 1992 to coincide with the United Nations Environmental Conference in South America and has been instrumental in helping to raise consciousness of the connection between food, agriculture, and the environment. This new edition, enlarged by over 50 percent, includes a wealth of new information, including the opening chapter on the legacy of Chief Seattle and Native American principles of balance; a new yin/yang analysis of the buildup of atmospheric carbon dioxide and other greenhouse gases; updated data, health statistics, and economic trends; and more practical steps that the ordinary individual or family can take to restore balance.

Healing Planet Earth is indispensable reading for every person on our planet. By taking responsibility for our own way of life, including way of eating, we can reverse the trend toward ecological destruction and bequeath a world of health and happiness to our children and grandchildren.

Alex Jack
Becket, Massachusetts
February 6, 1996

Alex Jack is director of One Peaceful World, a teacher at the Kushi Institute, and author of Out of Thin Air: A Satire on Owls & Ozone, Beef & Biodiversity, Grains & Global Warming *(One Peaceful World Press, 1993)*

Part One
Chief Seattle's Environmental Teachings

"When we talk about preservation of the environment, it is related to many other things. Ultimately the decision must come from the human heart. The key point is to have a genuine sense of universal responsibility, based on love and compassion, and clear awareness."—The Dalai Lama

Chief Seal'th, known today as Chief Seattle, lived in the forests and by the waters of Puget Sound. Seal'th was born around 1786 and died in 1866. He was a man of peace, wisdom, and far-reaching vision. In 1855 he signed a treaty which granted the white settlers ownership of the tribal lands of the Duwamish people. The city that grew on the Duwamish lands was named Seattle, in honor of the great chief.

In 1854, Chief Seattle gave a speech to territorial governor Isaac Stevens in which he presented his views on the surrender of his ancestral lands. His speech was recorded and edited several years later. Although the language may have been polished somewhat, the written text contains ideas that are fundamental to the Native American view of life. Chief Seattle's speech includes an eloquent description of humanity's relation to the earth, other forms of life, and the invisible world of spirit. Like the Tao Teh Ching, the Heart Sutra, and the Sermon on the Mount, it contains universal truths. In this remarkable statement, Chief Seattle reveals timeless wisdom. He includes a prophetic vision of modern environmental destruction, and offers future generations a blueprint for living in harmony with the earth. Below are excerpts from Chief Seattle's speech, which I have organized into passages followed by commentary.

> How can you buy or sell the sky, the warmth of the land? The idea is strange to us.
> If we do not own the freshness of the air and the sparkle of the water, how can you buy them?

The above lines, which read like *haiku*, are the product of a view of life that is the opposite of our own. For Chief Seattle, and countless traditional people before him, human life was understood to be the product of the earth, sky, sun, water, and air. Nature was seen as the common source of our existence. Nature created man; man did not create nature. Heaven and earth were here long before human beings arrived, and will be here long after our civilization has vanished. Such common sense existed in all traditional cultures, for example, in Ecclesiastes it states: "One generation passeth away, and another generation cometh; but the earth abideth forever."

Chief Seattle saw the world as an indivisible whole, a unified field, that could not be divided and parceled out. He saw his people, and all people, as beneficiaries of the natural abundance of the earth. He believed each generation had the responsibility to preserve that abundance and pass it on to future generations. The notion that something so common, essential, and priceless could be assigned monetary value, was, for him, beyond reason or comprehension. To Chief Seattle, human beings were temporary stewards of the earth, not the permanent owners of it.

> Every part of this earth is sacred to my people.
> Every shining pine needle, every sandy shore, every mist in the dark woods, every clearing and humming insect is holy in the memory

and experience of my people. The sap which courses through the trees carries the memories of the red man.

The white man's dead forget the country of their birth when they go to walk among the stars. Our dead never forget this beautiful earth, for it is the mother of the red man.

We are part of the earth and it is part of us.

The perfumed flowers are our sisters; the deer, the horse, the great eagle, these are our brothers.

The rocky crests, the juices in the meadows, the body heat of the pony, and man—all belong to the same family.

In the above passage, Chief Seattle describes humanity's unity with nature. Through countless centuries, the earth has left an invisible imprint on humanity, and humanity has in turn transferred its consciousness and spirit to the earth. Chief Seattle contrasts the unity his people felt for the earth with modern society's alienation from nature. He employs a spiritual metaphor to highlight the difference between these opposite ways of life, stating that when they die, civilized people "forget the country of their birth." In contrast, the ancestors of his people are a living presence: their spirit can be felt in the trees, streams, clouds, and wind. To respect the earth is to respect one's ancestors. To respect the earth is also to respect the source of our existence. Chief Seattle's teaching that "we are part of the earth and the earth is part of us" is the same as the Oriental concept of *Shin-do-fu-ji*, or "humanity and the earth are not two."

Chief Seattle and other traditional people saw all things in nature as manifestations of a universal spirit. In the closing lines, Chief Seattle affirms our kinship with the earth, stating that plants, animals, rocks, and humans are all part of one family.

So, when the Great Chief in Washington sends word that he wishes to buy our land, he asks

9

much of us. The Great Chief sends word he will reserve us a place so that we can live comfortably to ourselves.

He will be our father and we will be his children. So we will consider your offer to buy our land.

But it will not be easy. For this land is sacred to us.

This shining water that moves in the streams and rivers is not just water but the blood of our ancestors.

If we sell you land, you must remember that it is sacred, and you must teach your children that it is sacred and that each ghostly reflection in the clear water of the lakes tells of events and memories in the life of my people.

The water's murmur is the voice of my father's father.

In reading these lines, one feels the sadness and sense of loss Chief Seattle felt at the surrender of his ancestral lands. As a man of vision, Chief Seattle could see that modern civilization had become unstoppable. As a man of peace, he accepted the offer of the "Great Chief" without resistance. And, as a man of highly developed understanding, he placed spiritual rather than material conditions on the surrender of his land, by asking that future generations be taught to appreciate the invisible spirit of the land and treat it with the appropriate love, care, and respect. Modern environmental awareness is nothing but a reflection of Chief Seattle's spirit. Chief Seattle's vision continues to inspire millions of people and thus, the defeat which the surrender of his land represented could easily change into a lasting victory.

The rivers are our brothers, they quench our thirst. The rivers carry our canoes, and feed our children. If we sell you our land, you must remember, and teach your children, that the rivers are our brothers, and yours, and you must henceforth give the rivers the kindness you would give any brother.

We know that the white man does not understand our ways. One portion of land is the same to him as the next, for he is a stranger who comes in the night and takes from the land whatever he needs.

The earth is not his brother, but his enemy, and when he has conquered it, he moves on.

He leaves his father's graves behind, and he does not care. He kidnaps the earth from his children, and he does not care.

His father's grave, and his children's birthright, are forgotten. He treats his mother, the earth, and his brother, the sky, as things to be bought, plundered, sold like sheep or bright beads.

His appetite will devour the earth and leave behind only a desert.

I do not know. Our ways are different from your ways.

The sight of your cities pains the eyes of the red man. But perhaps it is because the red man is savage and does not understand.

There is no quiet place in the white man's cities.

No place to hear the unfurling of leaves in spring, or the rustle of an insect's wings.

But perhaps it is because I am a savage and do not understand.

The clatter only seems to insult the ears. And what is there to life if a man cannot hear the lonely cry of the whippoorwill or the arguments of the frogs around a pond at night? I am a red man and do not understand.

The Indian prefers the soft sound of the wind darting over the face of a pond, and the smell of the wind itself, cleaned by a midday rain, or scented with the pinion pine.

Chief Seattle opens the above passage by asking future generations to preserve the purity of the earth's waters. Water is essential to life, and Chief Seattle asks that the rivers (and other bodies of water) be treated with the kindness and respect one would extend to the members of one's family. He laments the spiritual blindness of modern civilization, stating that modern people, rather than seeking harmony with nature, seem to be at war with it. Chief Seattle's observation that when modern people have conquered the earth, they move on, accurately describes what is occurring today in tropical rain forests and other parts of the world. By plundering the environment, civilized man is separating himself from his past and future: he is squandering the inheritance received from his ancestors, while stealing the inheritance of future generations.

Chief Seattle then suggests that modern materialistic appetites could lead to destruction of the earth's biosphere, leaving behind nothing but a lifeless desert. Chief Seattle naturally found such a self-destructive tendency difficult to comprehend.

His prophecies are now coming true. In many parts of the world, modern agriculture, including the overgrazing of livestock, is depleting the earth's natural resources and turning fertile farmland into desert. Global deforestation, including destruction of tropical rain forests, could alter the earth's climate and lead to a wave of plant and animal extinction not seen since the disappearance of the dinosaurs over sixty million years ago. If not reversed, these trends could indeed turn the earth into a lifeless desert.

By using the image of a city filled with mechanical noise, Chief Seattle predicted modern civilization's increasing alienation from the natural world. Moreover, by suggesting that the expansion of civilization could result in the disappearance of birds, amphibians, and other species, he was envisioning the growing threat to biodiversity that has occurred in the 20th century. In *Silent Spring*, the classic book on the environment that alerted the world to the dangers posed by DDT and other pesticides, Rachel Carson cited numerous cases showing a decline in the population of birds following chemical spraying of farms and forests:

> Over increasingly large areas of the United States, spring now comes unheralded by the return of the birds, and early mornings are strangely silent where once they were filled with the beauty of bird song. This sudden silencing of the song of birds, this obliteration of the color and beauty and interest they lend to our world have come about swiftly, insidiously, and unnoticed by those whose communities are as yet unaffected.

The use of pesticides has not decreased since publication of *Silent Spring* in 1962. A Greenpeace report released on the 30th anniversary of Rachel Carson's book found that in the last generation global sales of pesticides have increased 31 times. Approximately 4 billion pounds of pesticides are used worldwide every year. Two-thirds of the dangerous chemicals highlighted in *Silent Spring* are still manufactured and used around the world. According to the World Health Organization, up to a million people are injured each year as a direct result of pesticide exposure or ingestion. The effect of pesticides is insidious and all-encompassing: in a survey of 38 states, the EPA found at least 74 pesticides in ground water. Meanwhile, in a perfect example of the law of compensation that governs the natural world, more than 650 species of weeds and insects have become resistant to chemical sprays.

In his book *The Diversity of Life*, Harvard biologist Edward O. Wilson points to another cause of the decline of birds in North America:

> From the 1940s to the 1980s, population densities of migratory songbirds in the mid-Atlantic United States dropped 50 percent, and many species became locally extinct. One cause appears to be the accelerating destruction of the forests of the West Indies, Mexico, and Central and South America, the principal wintering grounds of

13

many of the migrants. The fate of Bachman's warbler will probably befall many North American summer residents if the deforestation continues.

In the mid-1980s, biologists in the field began to notice a mysterious decline in populations of frogs, toads, and salamanders. Reports indicate that the disappearance of amphibians is worldwide, for example, at least one-third of the 86 frog and toad species in North America and 10 percent of the 194 species of frogs in Australia are currently in decline. Reductions of 50 percent or more have been noted in certain species. In some cases, outright local extinctions have occurred. Moreover, up to 33 percent of North America's fish are now rare or imperiled due to pollution, habitat destruction, and over-fishing. Meanwhile, in the vegetable world, 250 species of North American plants face possible extinction within the next five years. Biologists believe the decline in amphibian populations may be the result of humanity's disruption of the environment, including depletion of the ozone layer (many species of amphibians are highly sensitive to ultraviolet radiation) and destruction of their natural habitats.

Amphibians spend the early part of their life in ponds, streams, and other bodies of fresh water, after which they emerge from their aquatic environment and begin breathing air. They are sensitive to the condition of the earth's fresh waters and atmosphere, and thus mirror of the health of the environment as a whole. Biologists believe the disappearance of frogs and toads may be an early warning sign of some as yet unknown change in our planetary environment. If the decline in amphibian populations continues, humanity may no longer be able to enjoy the pleasure of hearing "the arguments of frogs around a pond at night," or be inspired to write a poem like the famous one by Basho:

Furuike ya, kawazu tobikomu, mizu no oto.

"Breaking the silence of an ancient pond,
A frog jumped into water—
A deep resonance."

The air is precious to the red man, for all things share the same breath—the beast, the tree, the man, they all share the same breath.

The white man does not seem to notice the air he breathes. Like a man dying for many days, he is numb to the stench.

But if we sell you our land, you must remember that the air is precious to us, that the air shares its spirit with all the life it supports. The wind that gave our grandfather his first breath also receives his last sigh.

And if we sell you our land, you must keep it apart and sacred, as a place where even the white man can go to taste the wind that is sweetened by the meadow's flowers.

Here Chief Seattle describes the importance of fresh clean air—the vital breath of life. He states that "air shares its spirit with all the life it supports." Like traditional people in both East and West, Chief Seattle viewed life in terms of energy or "spirit." In India, life energy was referred to as *prana*. Practices such as yoga, breathing, and meditation aim at developing life energy, and are referred to in Sanskrit as *pranayama*.

People in China and Japan referred to the energy of life as *ch'i* or *ki*. An understanding of life energy is part of the everyday life of people in Asia where both human and natural phenomena are referred to as manifestations of *ki*. In Japanese, for example, air is called *ku-ki*, or the "energy of emptiness." Weather is known as *ten-ki*, or the "energy of heaven," and electricity is called *den-ki*, or the "energy of thunder." Courage is known as *yu-ki*, or "active energy," and cowardice is referred to as *ki-ga-chisai*," or "energy is small." Like Native Americans and other indigenous peoples, people in the Far East saw all things as manifestations of energy or spirit.

For thousands of years, the understanding of energy has provided the basis for the healing arts and spiritual practices of the Orient. In China and Japan, energy was understood to flow through clearly defined lines or meridians, along which numerous points are located. In India, energy was understood to flow deep within the body along a vertical channel from the top of the head to the sexual organs. There are seven highly charged energy centers located along the vertical channel, all of which supply the internal organs and functions. These energy centers, or chakras, are also the source of thought, image, and consciousness. The meridians originate within the primary channel and chakras, radiate out toward the periphery of the body, and return to the chakras. Energy moves from center to periphery and periphery to center in a continuous cycle.

The meridian network runs just below the skin. Each meridian continuously subdivides into countless tiny branches, which Michio Kushi has named "meridian branches." Each branch ends in a cell. Each of the body's cells is thus provided with invisible life energy through the meridians and their branches, and with physical nutrients through the bloodstream. Each part of the body is linked with all the others through the meridian network. What happens in one part of the body affects all the other parts.

The earth also has an invisible energy form through which all of its parts are linked. The earth's energy form parallels that of the human body. The highly charged aurora borealis, or Northern lights, radiating above the North Pole, corresponds to the human aura surrounding the head. Energy radiates outward from the core of the earth in the same way it radiates outward from the chakras to form meridians. The earth's meridians are its mountain ranges. Michio Kushi and I describe the differentiation of the earth's meridians in the book, *Other Dimensions*:

> Branching off from the earth's mountain ranges, or meridians, are invisible lines of energy that form a sort of power grid on the planet's surface. Ancient people tracked these invisible pathways and often cleared the land above them. These manmade tracks, called ley lines (from the Saxon word for "meadow" or "cleared strip of land"), correspond to the streams of energy that branch

16

off from the body's meridians. They also link megalithic structures such as Stonehenge and have been found throughout the British Isles, Europe, and the Andes. In western Bolivia, these lines are called *ta-kis,* which means "spirit paths." Interestingly, the word "ki" was used by the ancient Andeans to describe energy or spirit just as it was used by the Japanese.

These invisible streams continuously subdivide, linking all of the earth's geological features in an invisible network. Every rock, river, mountain, and valley is part of the earth's energy grid. The energy of the earth is in turn transferred to plants and animals. Earth's force interacts with celestial energy to produce and animate all life on earth. The environment is a unified system, an organic whole, linked by invisible streams of energy. Nothing exists in isolation. As a result, environmental disruption can never be limited to one place. Disruption of the environment in one part of the world produces a series of reactions that reverberate throughout the environment as a whole, in the same way that sickness in one part of the body affects all the others. Each part influences the whole; the whole influences each part. Compensation, or action and reaction, is the operating principle of the natural world.

The passage closes with Chief Seattle's plea to keep the air unspoiled and pure, so that future generations will be able to "taste the wind that is sweetened by the meadow's flowers."

So we will accept your offer to buy our land. If we decide to accept, I will make one condition. The white man must treat the beasts of this land as his brothers.

I am a savage and I do not understand any other way.

I have seen a thousand rotting buffaloes on the prairie, left by the white man who shot them from a passing train.

I am a savage and I do not understand how

the smoking iron horse can be more important than the buffalo that we kill only to stay alive.

What is man without the beasts? If all the beasts were gone, man would die from a great loneliness of spirit.

For whatever happens to the beasts happens to man. All things are connected.

The above passage contains an eloquent plea for preserving the rich diversity of life on earth. Chief Seattle links the preservation of biodiversity to the very survival of the human spirit. The wholesale slaughter of the buffalo, whose herds once stretched from the Appalachians to the Rockies, was a potent symbol of environmental destruction in the last century. Like the destruction of tropical rain forests today, the slaughter of the buffalo was prompted by industrial, banking, and ranching interests intent on turning the Great Plains into a vast cattle preserve. Today, the production of livestock utilizes an area of land equivalent to about half the continental United States for feed crops, pasture, and range. The destruction of the buffalo is thus a symbol for the rise of the cattle culture and the increasing reliance on meat and dairy food in the diet.

In stating that "whatever happens to the beasts, soon happens to man," Chief Seattle reveals an understanding of the law of karma, compensation, or cause and effect. The slaughter of the buffalo in the 19th century led to an explosion in the cattle population of North America and to increasing consumption of meat and dairy. Increasing consumption of animal food has, in turn, produced a catastrophic rise in the incidence of cancer, heart disease, and other degenerative diseases in the 20th century. The wheel of karma spins without end. What goes around comes around. The fate that has befallen the beasts is now befalling modern man.

Chief Seattle understood that the way in which we relate to our outer environment is a reflection of our inner environment, or our health and thinking. Modern civilization's mistreatment of the environment is thus a product of widespread physical, mental, and spiritual disorder.

You must teach your children that the ground beneath their feet is the ashes of your grandfathers. So that they will respect the land, tell your children that the earth is rich with the lives of our kin.

Teach your children what we have taught our children, that the earth is our mother.

Whatever befalls the earth, befalls the sons of the earth. If men spit upon the ground, they spit upon themselves.

This we know: The earth does not belong to man; man belongs to the earth. This we know.

All things are connected like the blood which unites one family. All things are connected.

Whatever befalls the earth befalls the sons of the earth. Man did not weave the web of life; he is merely a strand in it. Whatever he does to the web, he does to himself.

Even the white man, whose God walks and talks with him as friend to friend, cannot be exempt from the common destiny.

We may be brothers after all.

We shall see.

One thing we know, which the white man may one day discover—our God is the same God.

You may think now that you own Him as you wish to own our land; but you cannot. He is the God of man, and his compassion is equal for the red man and the white.

This earth is precious to Him, and to harm the earth is to heap contempt on its Creator.

The whites too shall pass; perhaps sooner than all other tribes. Contaminate your bed, and you will one night suffocate in your own waste.

But in your perishing you will shine brightly, fired by the strength of the God who brought you to this land and for some special purpose gave you dominion over this land and over the red man.

That destiny is a mystery to us, for we do not understand when the buffalo are all slaughtered, the wild horses are tamed, the secret corners of the forest are heavy with the scent of many men, and the view of the ripe hills blotted by talking wires.

Where is the thicket? Gone.

Where is the eagle? Gone.

The end of living and the beginning of survival.

The above lines contain the essence of Chief Seattle's teachings on life, nature, and humanity. The passage begins with the basic truth that human life is intimately connected to the soil. The earth carries the spirit of past generations, and should be treated with the appropriate care and respect. The earth is also the source, or mother of life, and the health of the planet is equivalent to the health of humanity. If we contaminate our environment, we contaminate ourselves. It is sobering to realize that the United States produces 700,000 tons of hazardous waste every day. Americans are now exposed to more than 65,000 synthetic chemicals, with another 10,000 added each year.

Chief Seattle describes the interconnectedness of creation in terms of the "web" of life. A spider's web is actually a spiral, and Chief Seattle employed a spiral image to describe the pattern of creation. The spiral is the one universal form found throughout nature. Using the image of a spiral, we can see that the earth is a tiny ephemeral point within the unchanging ocean of infinity. Creation occurs in the form of an inward, contracting spiral and begins with the polarization of one infinity into two complementary and antagonistic forces, or yin and yang. The two poles produce energy, or vibrations, and these condense into electrons, protons, and other preatomic particles. The combination of preatomic particles results in the creation of atoms and elements. The plant world is the product of the elements, or the world of nature. The plant kingdom gives rise to the world of animals, and ultimately, human beings. The creation of the universe occurs in the form of a spiral with seven orbits or stages.

The Web of Life

1. God or One Infinity
2. Heaven and Earth
3. Energy and Vibration
4. Subatomic Particles
5. Elements and Compounds
6. Vegetable Kingdom
7. Animal Kingdom culminating with Human Beings

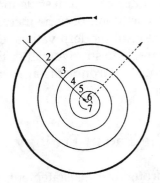

Chief Seattle presents several truths that follow from his understanding of the spiral of life. The first is that everything is connected, and everything shares the same universal source: "All things are connected like the blood which unites one family." Humanity, nature, and the universe are all strands within the web of life. The second is that man is the product of nature, and not vice-versa: "The earth does not belong to man; man belongs to the earth." Humanity did not create the spiral of life, but is only one small manifestation of it. Chief Seattle also suggests that man's inner world—his body and mind—and his outer world, which is made up of spiral of life, are one: "Man did not weave the web of life; he is merely a strand in it. Whatever he does to the web, he does to himself." Such an awareness of the relationship between personal and planetary destiny is fundamental to an ecological way of life.

To Chief Seattle, God, or the infinite universe is the same for everyone. All people and all things share the same origin and destiny. In that regard, all people are brothers and sisters of one infinite universe, and all are members of the planetary family of humanity. To respect the manifestations of God is to respect God. To disrespect them is to disrespect God. Because he understood that the process of change is eternal, Chief Seattle knew that all human works are ephemeral. All things shall pass. He clearly states that if modern civilization continues to predicate itself on the domination and destruction of nature, it shall pass sooner rather than later.

Chief Seattle's final prophecy was meant for future generations: should destruction of the environment continue, life on earth will become increasingly harsh and difficult. Unless and until modern values undergo a fundamental change, the struggle to survive, rather than the freedom to enjoy our wondrous environment on earth, will remain the paramount issue.

The Tao of Ecology

Throughout his statement, Chief Seattle contrasts the way of his people with the way of modern civilization. Native Americans were living as a part of nature, not separate from it. Their natural lifestyle was not unlike Lao Tsu's ideal of living according to the Tao. The Tao is the way of nature, the way of the universe. Chief Seattle's people were living close to nature with a minimum of artificiality and waste.

Lao Tsu lived 2,500 years before Chief Seattle. In the Tao Teh Ching, one of the greatest philosophical classics of all time, Lao Tsu describes the difference between the natural and artificial:

> When what is natural [the Tao] prevails in human affairs, horses forced to train for racing are returned to the fertile pastures. When artificiality prevails in human affairs, horses are trained for war and are restricted to walled enclosures.

When the Tao is practiced in society, humanity co-exists peacefully with the environment. People cooperate with nature, rather than seeking to conquer, "improve," or destroy it. Lao Tsu taught "non-doing," or non-interference with the way of nature. Humanity did not create Tao. Tao created the earth, humanity, and all living beings. The Tao (nature) is infinitely vast and powerful, and humanity, as an infinitesimally small manifestation of Tao, must learn how to adapt to and live in harmony with it. Respect for the natural environment is one of the first steps in the healing process.

Contained within the understanding of Tao are the seeds of a truly ecological way of living. The Tao is wholeness itself. To live in accord with Tao means that we balance—both in ourselves and our surroundings—the opposite forces that comprise wholeness. The way of Tao is thus the way of health and healing. The English words "health" and "healing" come from the same root as the word "whole." Health or wholeness result from harmony between yin and yang, the opposite yet complementary forces that govern the natural world, including our existence as human beings. The key to achieving health and wholeness can be found in the root of the English word medicine. The word "medicine" comes from the Latin root, *medire*, or "to walk in the middle." The middle way is the way in which we avoid extremes, harmonizing and balancing yin and yang in all aspects of life.

In the Tao Teh Ching, Lao Tsu offers a hint for solving the modern crisis in personal and planetary health:

> Nip troubles in the bud. Sow the great in the small. Difficult things of the world can only be tackled when they are easy. Big things of the world can only be achieved by attending to their small beginnings.

In order to solve the crisis in personal and global health, we need to adopt Chief Seattle's and Lao Tsu's spirit and way of thinking as our own. On a practical level, we need a planetary medicine that we can apply in daily life. The new planetary medicine should be able to help us solve problems of personal health as well as problems of a global scale. It must be accessible to everyone.

The root of the environmental crisis lies in each of us—in our hearts, our minds, and our daily way of life. The solution to a problem as large and seemingly complex as the fate of life on earth may actually be quite simple. As Lao Tsu said, it is easy to solve problems when they are small. Healing the earth begins with us. In the pages that follow, we explore the ways in which our dietary and lifestyle choices influence not only our own health and the health of our families, but the health of our planetary environment and the quality of life of future generations.

Part Two
Diet and the New Ecology

"There is no drop of water in the ocean, not even in the deepest parts of the abyss, that does not know and respond to the mysterious forces that create the tide."
—Rachel Carson

In August 1992, Bill Clinton received the Democratic Party's nomination for president. Soon afterward, I wrote to him (on One Peaceful World stationery) about the macrobiotic approach to personal health and the environment:

> One behalf of those in the macrobiotic, natural food, environmental, and holistic health movements, I congratulate you on being selected as the Democratic Party's candidate for president, and on your choice of Albert Gore as your running mate. I appreciate Senator Gore's strong stand on environmental issues and his commitment to a cleaner and healthier planet.
>
> For the past thirty years, my associates and I have been working to promote awareness of an ecologically balanced diet. It is my firm belief that an environmentally sound lifestyle begins with the selection of whole natural foods. Under the name of macrobiotics, millions of people throughout the world have begun to eat a natural, eco-

logically balanced diet based on whole cereal grains, fresh local vegetables, and other products of regional, non-polluting, and self-sustaining agriculture.

Evidence is accumulating that a diet based on these foods may be of enormous benefit to personal health. The basic principles of macrobiotics—for example, reducing the intake of high-fat animal food, sugar, and refined foods, and basing the diet on whole grains, beans, and fresh local vegetables—have been endorsed by the United States Senate in the landmark 1977 report, *Dietary Goals for the United States*; by the National Academy of Sciences in the 1982 report, *Diet, Nutrition and Cancer*; by the U.S. Surgeon General in the 1988 report, *Diet and Health*; and by reports issued by other scientific and public health agencies in the United States and abroad. Around the world, a consensus is building that a naturally balanced diet along the lines of macrobiotics would substantially reduce the incidence of chronic disease.

In his State of the Union address, President Bush announced that medical costs in the United States reached $800 billion in 1991, and will climb to a staggering $1.6 trillion by the year 2000. I firmly believe that the continuing escalation of medical costs will severely disrupt the world economy by the early part of the next century. The economic benefit of reducing the number of chronic diseases in the United States would be tremendous. Given our current situation, the need for preventive health strategies, including proper diet, has never been more urgent.

Not only is the modern diet a primary cause of the rising incidence of chronic disease, it is also a major contributor to the continuing degradation of the environment. The modern food system is based on the inefficient conversion of foods such as cereal grains and beans into animal protein and fat, in the form of meat, chicken, milk, cheese, butter, and eggs. Modern agriculture and food processing waste a tremendous amount of energy, largely in the form of fossil fuels. The burning of fossil fuels by various segments of the food industry contributes a great deal of carbon dioxide to the atmosphere, and is a primary contributor to global warming.

It is far more efficient to eat plant foods directly. Whole grains, beans, fresh local vegetables, sea vegetables and other foods produced by regional organic agriculture are far more energy-efficient than modern beef, chicken, and other forms of animal food.

Destruction of the rain forest is linked to the modern diet. As you may know, cattle ranching is a leading cause of tropical deforestation. According to Edward O. Wilson, 55,000 square miles of rain forest (an area larger than the state of Florida) disappears every year. The wholesale destruction of such a precious natural resource would be substantially reduced if America shifted toward a grain- and vegetable-based diet.

I would be happy to discuss these issues in person with you or with Senator Gore. I would like to hear your views and those of Senator Gore about the possibility of focusing public attention on the role of diet in personal and planetary health, and the possibility of reducing medical costs by implementing preventive strategies that incorporate a naturally balanced diet.

Several weeks later, I received a courteous reply in which Governor Clinton thanked me for "information about One Peaceful World and a healthful diet," and mentioned that he and Al Gore appreciated my encouragement. Unfortunately, however, as the summer changed into autumn, and the election drew closer, our meeting never came to pass. Perhaps my request got lost amidst the whirlwind of the presidential campaign or was overshadowed by other issues.

Earth in the Balance

In *Earth in the Balance*, his best-selling book on the environment, Vice President Al Gore characterizes the environmental crisis as an increasingly critical loss of balance. The book is divided into three sections, each of which incorporates the word balance in the title. The theme of balance is discussed throughout the book, beginning in the introduction:

> I have come therefore to believe that the world's ecological balance depends on more than just our ability to restore a balance between civilization's ravenous appetite for resources and the fragile equilibrium of the earth's environment; it depends on more even, than our ability to restore a balance between ourselves as individuals and the civilization we aspire to create and sustain. In the end we must restore a balance within ourselves between who we are and what we are doing. Each of us must take a greater personal responsibility for this deteriorating global environment; each of us must take a hard look at the habits of mind and action that reflect—and have led to—this grave crisis.

The issue of balance is also taken up in the concluding chapter:

> Perhaps because I have ended up searching simultaneously for a better understanding of my own life and of what can be done to rescue the global environment, I have come to believe in the value of a kind of inner ecology that relies on the same principles of balance and holism that characterize a healthy environment. The key is indeed

balance—balance between contemplation and action, individual concerns and commitment to the community, love for the natural world and love for our wondrous civilization. This is the balance I seek in my own life.

The modern crisis in personal and planetary health is indeed a crisis of balance. But what is balance and how can we restore it? Webster's defines balance as "equipoise between contrasting, opposing, or interacting elements." Balance is therefore equivalent to the harmony of opposites, for example, between movement and rest, heat and cold, production and consumption, carbon and oxygen, forest and desert, rainfall and dryness, taking in and discharging, sound and silence, activity and reflection.

We live in a universe comprised of complementary opposites. Our body, for example, has a front and a back; the front is soft and expanded, and the back, hard and condensed. We have a left and a right side that work together in a complementary harmony. The body has a center and a periphery, and parts that are hidden and parts that are visible. The body also has a top and a bottom, or an upper region and a lower one. When taken together, these complementary opposites comprise the unity of our existence.

All complementary opposites are actually different appearances of two primal forces. Physical attributes such as temperature, size, weight, structure, form, position, and direction of movement yield numerous complementary tendencies that display a stronger tendency either toward expansive force, or toward contractive force. Thousands of years ago, these primary forces were given the names yin and yang. Yin refers to the primary force of expansion (centrifugal force) found throughout nature. Yang refers to the primary force of contraction (centripetal force). Although the terms yin and yang were first used in China, a similar concept can be found in all traditional cultures. The principle of yin and yang provides a universal compass that can help us find and maintain balance under any circumstances. It is the key to achieving balance within ourselves and with our planetary environment.

On the following page, we classify a variety of complementary attributes into yin and yang. There are many ways to classify things into complementary categories, and the chart presented below represents only one way based on the definition of yin and yang described above. Yin and yang are not absolutes, if anything, they are absolutely relative. All things are composed of both of these forces, and nothing is entirely yin or entirely yang. Moreover, things are not yin or yang of themselves, but only in relation to other things. Let us consider a few examples.

When things expand (yin), they increase in size, and when they contract (yang), they become smaller. Largeness is created by expansion, and smallness, by contraction. Expanding force tends to push things toward the outside, or periphery, while contracting force causes them to gather toward the center. Upward motion is actually a form of expanding motion away from the earth, while downward movement is a form of contracting motion toward the earth. Largeness, upward motion, and a peripheral (outside) position are produced by expansion and are yin. Smallness, downward motion, and a central (inside) position are created by contracting force and are yang.

Using expansion and contraction as our reference points, we can classify many other complementary attributes into either of these categories. For example, if something has a predominantly vertical form, a greater portion of its mass extends upward away from the earth. If something has a predominantly horizontal form, a greater portion of its mass lies closer to the earth. Upward, or yin movement gives rise to vertical forms, while yang downward movement produces horizontal forms. Wetness and dryness can also be understood in terms of yin and yang. When seeds absorb water, for example, they become larger, and when they dry out, they contract and shrink. Wetness is thus yin, and dryness, yang.

Expansion causes atoms and molecules to separate, making things become lighter and less dense. Contraction bunches atoms and molecules together, thus making things become dense and heavy. Density and heaviness can thus be grouped

Examples of Yin and Yang

	YIN	YANG
	Centrifugal force	**Centripetal force**
General Tendency	Expansion	Contraction
Function	Diffusion	Fusion
Movement	More inactive, slower	More active and faster
Vibration	Shorter wave and high frequency	Longer wave and low frequency
Direction	Ascent and vertical	Descent and horizontal
Position	More outward and periphery	More inward and central
Weight	Lighter	Heavier
Temperature	Colder	Hotter
Light	Darker	Brighter
Humidity	Wetter	Drier
Density	Thinner	Thicker
Size	Longer	Smaller
Shape	More expansive and fragile	More contractive and harder
Atomic particle	Electron	Proton
Elements	N,O, K, P, Ca, etc.	H, C, Na, As, Mg, etc.
Environment	Vibration...Air...Water...	Earth
Climatic effects	Tropical climate	Colder climate
Biological	More vegetable quality	More animal quality
Sex	Female	Male
Organ structure	More hollow and expansive	More compacted and condensed
Attitude	More gentle, negative	More active, positive
Work	More psychological and mental	More physical and social
Dimension	Space	Time

with the attributes on the right, while lightness can be classified with the attributes on the left. Solids are usually denser and heavier than liquids and gases, and the solid state can be included with the yang characteristics in the right-hand column. Liquids and gases are lighter and more diffuse. The liquid and gaseous states thus match the other yin attributes in the left-hand column.

Heat is a property of contracting force or movement. Cold is created by expansion. Space, which expands infinitely in all directions, is cold, while heat is a product of stars and planets, which are condensed material forms. Space is also dark. Brightness is a characteristic of the condensed points known as stars. Therefore, heat and brightness can be classified with the other characteristics in the column on the right, while coldness and darkness match the attributes on the left.

Our environment on earth is a masterpiece of balance. Space is yin or expanded, while in comparison, the earth is tiny, solid, and yang. However, even though it has a yin form, the universe produces movement in the form of contracting spirals, similar to the way that cold (also yin) causes things to contract. Energy from the universe spirals inward and condenses. As it makes the transition from energy to matter, it creates preatomic particles and atoms, leading to the formation of stars, planets, and solid objects.

Heaven's force appears on the earth as a contractive, centripetal, or downward force (yang) that pushes everything toward the surface of the planet. The earth, because of its rotation, gives off a stream of expansive, centrifugal, or upward force (yin). Together these forces create the wide range of environments on our planet, from mountain ranges to flat plains, from deserts to tropical forests, and from small volcanic islands to vast continents.

Northern regions with cold climates are yin, and make balance with hot southern areas. However, low temperatures produce slow, contracted growth, which is yang, while high temperatures produce rapid, expanded, and lush growth, which is yin. The plants and animals in tropical areas are thus yin, while those in the polar or temperate zones are yang.

Moist environments, such as those near a river or lake,

are yin, while deserts and other dry places are yang. Sodium is a yang element, and islands, which are surrounded by salt water, are yang, as are coastal areas. In comparison, continental environments are yin. Mountains are formed by upward energy, and are yin, while valleys and plains are formed by downward force and are yang. The classification of environments into yin and yang is summarized below.

Complementary Environments

Yin	Yang
Colder, northern	Warmer, southern
Humid	Dry
Continent	Island
Mountainous	Flat
Inland	Coastal
Near lakes or rivers	More arid or desert
Forest	Plains or fields
Rich in vegetation	Rocky or sandy
Rural	Urban
Low-tech	High-tech

The environment in the city is more yang than that in the country for a number of reasons. Vegetation is created largely by the expanding or yin energy of the earth. It is plentiful in the country. The urban environment is made up of concrete, steel, and glass. Industry and technology, which are based on the use of fire or energy, create yang energy, and are prevalent in an urban environment. Industrial activities release carbon dioxide, metals, and positive ions, all of which are yang. The air in the country is clearer, richer in oxygen, and contains a higher number of negative ions.

Researchers conducting worldwide surveys have found that in rural areas, the concentration of metals in the environment resulting from industrial activity is between 10 and 100 times greater than in the remote North Atlantic. In cities, the concentrations are between 100 and 10,000 times greater. The dense population in the city is yang in relation to the sparse population of the country. According to the U.S. Census Bureau, there are 2,000 people per square mile in urban areas; while in rural areas, there are eighteen. All in all, the concentration of energy, activity, and people makes the environment in the city more yang than that in the country.

Nature Recycles

Yin and yang are not static, but dynamically moving and changing. Day changes into night, and night changes into day. The seasons change in a repeating cycle. All in all, the earth maintains a beautiful, moving harmony between numerous complementary opposites. The dynamic balance between heat and cold is but one example.

The ocean at the equator is constantly heated by the sun's rays. Heat, which is yang, produces expansion, or yin. Yin, expanded ocean water rises toward the surface, while the strong charge of centrifugal force at the equator causes it to radiate toward the poles. This is how the Gulf Stream and other warm water currents originate. When these currents reach the Far North, they encounter cold air. In the inverse of what occurs at the equator, cold, which is yin, produces contraction, or yang. Yang energy causes the warm ocean currents to become denser and heavier. This strongly yang water has a higher concentration of salt and rapidly sinks to the bottom at the rate of five billion gallons each second. The predominance of centripetal force at the poles causes deep currents, which are as powerful as the Gulf Stream, to form above the ocean floor. These cold water currents flow from the poles to to the equator. In this way, heat is distributed toward the poles, and cold moves toward the equator, creating the overall balance of the earth's climate.

The flow of heat and cold in the oceans offers an example of yin changing into yang and yang changing into yin. Elements continually cycle through the biosphere in a similar way. The nitrogen cycle, which is vital to life, is an example. Nitrogen continually cycles back and forth between yang and yin, or contraction and expansion, downward and upward movement, solidification and diffusion. In its yin form, nitrogen exists as a gas. Gaseous nitrogen forms more than 70 percent of the earth's atmosphere. Bacteria, fungi, and algae convert nitrogen into a solid form and provide it to plants for their growth and development.

Symbiotic bacteria live within the root systems of plants and receive nutrients from the plant tissues in exchange for providing the plant with nitrate, which for the bacteria, is a waste product. Symbiotic relationships occur everywhere in nature and are an example of the attraction and harmony that exist between yin and yang.

Nitrate is used by the plant to form amino acids, proteins, nucleic acids, and other compounds. These processes comprise the yang portion of the cycle. In the yin portion, plants die and bacteria decompose these compounds back into atmospheric nitrogen. When animals or humans eat plants, they discharge nitrogen compounds through excretion. Through a series of biochemical processes, bacteria break these organic residues down into their basic components, including atmospheric nitrogen, and the cycle begins again. Similar cycles govern the movement of water, carbon, and other elements in our environment. The movement of solar energy through the biosphere is another example.

The Transformation of Solar Energy

All life depends on the energy of the sun. In its most diffused, or yin state, matter exists in the form of plasma, or free electrons and protons. Upon reaching the most expanded stage, a process of condensation occurs, in which these preatomic particles bond with one another, eventually forming atoms. As the contracting process continues, atoms bond with each other, forming molecules, and matter begins to assume a definite form. Upon reaching a condensed solid state, matter then begins to expand, passing through the stages of liquid and gas, and ultimately returning to plasma, at which time the cycle begins again.

The process in which solar energy is stored by plants and converted by humans and animals into cellular energy follows a similar pattern. In this cycle, we can trace the transformation of energy through the following stages:

Solar Energy The earth receives about 1,000 watts of solar energy per square yard per minute, mostly in the form of light and heat. Most of the energy received by the earth is either reflected back into space or absorbed by the earth's surface and re-radiated as heat. The sun is an example of the plasma state of matter, as are stars, nebulae, galaxies, and practically all of the matter in the universe.

Photosynthesis During photosynthesis, solar energy is absorbed by green plants and combined with carbon dioxide and water to produce carbohydrates. Photosynthesis is a yang process in which free energy is condensed or stored, and uses less than 1 percent of the solar energy received by the earth. It is a product of the influence of sunlight on water molecules composed of hydrogen and oxygen. Sunlight, which is yang, is readily absorbed by yin oxygen atoms, causing them to become yang and thus less attracted to hydrogen atoms which are also yang. As the bonds holding the water molecule together weaken, the molecule breaks apart. Oxygen is released into the atmosphere and hydrogen combines with carbon dioxide to form glucose.

Glucose is the first type of food made by green plants, and all other types of vegetable food, including proteins, are the result of chemical alterations of this basic organic compound. The potential energy stored in glucose is the primary source of the biological energy that nourishes all living things. Modern civilization is also dependent on the potential energy of glucose, since most of the energy used to drive our automobiles, heat our homes, and power our appliances can be traced to this source.

Biosynthesis In the process known as biosynthesis, the sun's energy reaches its most concentrated, or yang state as the glucose produced by photosynthesis is stored in the form of complex polysaccharides. These large carbohydrate molecules are formed by the fusion of many small molecules of glucose, and exist in higher plants in the form of starch. In the rice plant, for example, each grain is composed mostly of starch in the form of polysaccharide glucose. The proteins, minerals, vitamins, and fats in brown rice are all built around polysaccharide glucose.

Digestion During digestion, energy begins moving in the opposite, or yin direction. When we eat grains and vegetables, for example, the molecules of complex carbohydrate created during biosynthesis are broken down into simple glucose. The breakdown of carbohydrates begins as soon as food enters the mouth. The polysaccharide glucose found in cereal grains, beans, and other plant foods is broken down largely in the mouth through the action of enzymes in saliva. Thorough chewing, which mixes food with saliva, is essential in releasing the potential energy contained in these foods. Man is unique among the animals in that, between the stages of biosynthesis and digestion, another process has been added. The additional process, cooking, can be considered as a form of pre-digestion, since it allows for the efficient breakdown and release of energy stored in plants. Cooked foods are more strongly energized than uncooked foods.

Respiration Through respiration, the energy stored in plants is converted back into energy and released. The release of energy (a yin process) occurs at the cellular level and the effect is the reverse of photosynthesis. Respiration requires oxygen, which is provided through breathing, and is the principal mechanism through which living things derive energy. Carbon dioxide and water, the elements used in photosynthesis, are given off as waste products. The end product of respiration is the conversion of glucose into free energy which is used by each of the body's cells.

Photosynthesis and biosynthesis are the stages in the biological energy cycle in which energy is condensed and stored, and are the product of yang, centripetal force. Digestion and respiration are the complementary processes through which energy is released, and are the product of yin centrifugal or expanding energy. Biological life exists on earth because of the dynamic exchange of yin and yang energies.

Our Changing Atmosphere

The rhythm that governs the tides, the phases of the moon, and the changing of the seasons can be seen in the atmosphere that surrounds the planet. When it is summer in the Northern Hemisphere, plant life becomes more abundant. Plants absorb carbon dioxide, which is yang, and discharge oxygen, which is yin. This causes the amount of carbon dioxide in the atmosphere to go down while the amount of oxygen increases. In the winter, when plant life becomes contracted and dormant, the amount of carbon dioxide increases and the amount of oxygen goes down. Since most of the earth's land area is in the Northern Hemisphere, these changes affect the atmosphere as a whole. Thus, the atmosphere becomes yin in summer and yang in winter.

Carbon and oxygen are strongly polarized: that is why they combine easily and form compounds such as carbon dioxide. Carbon dioxide makes up only .03 percent of the atmosphere by volume. Oxygen comprises about 21 percent and nitrogen about 78 percent. Because molecules of carbon dioxide contain an atom of carbon, they are more yang than molecules of oxygen. As we saw above, plants, which are yin, attract and absorb carbon dioxide. They also repel or discharge oxygen. Animals are yang, so they attract oxygen and repel carbon dioxide. The balance between carbon and oxygen is crucial to the balance of the environment as a whole.

Carbon exists in a multitude of forms. In its yin form, carbon exists as an invisible gas, carbon dioxide. Carbon also exists in a very yang form: literally the hardest substance that we know—a diamond. There are also a variety of in-between forms such as plants or coal or carbon powder. As we can see, carbon exists in many forms in various combinations and structures, some yin, others yang. In all of these different forms, we are still dealing with the same element, carbon.

Carbon is constantly in motion, cycling back and forth between yin and yang. It cycles through the atmosphere from the yin, invisible form of a gas, to yang visible forms, and back into the atmosphere again. During the yang part of the cycle, carbon dioxide is absorbed by plants, and is used to form the structure of the plant. Carbon is a primary ingredient in carbohydrates, proteins, and fats. During the yin part of the cycle, plants eventually die and decay, releasing carbon into the atmosphere. When animals eat plants, they convert their carbohydrates into energy and discharge carbon dioxide as waste. Carbon in the atmosphere cycles through plants, animals, and then back to atmosphere again in what can be called the "surface cycle" of carbon.

Natural Recycling

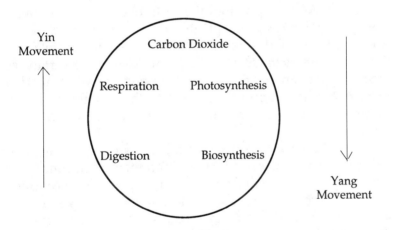

Through photosynthesis and biosynthesis, plants convert carbon dioxide into carbohydrates. Through digestion and respiration, animals convert carbohydrates into carbon dioxide and energy.

Plants, animals, and human beings have coexisted at the surface of the carbon cycle for millions of years, during which time there were no global threats to the environment caused by human activity. People ate whole grains, beans, and other energy-efficient complex carbohydrate foods directly, rather than passing them first through livestock, and used biomass, in the form of wood, straw, charcoal, and other plant-based materials, as their primary source of energy. Using carbon in these forms is clean and efficient. Eating complex carbohydrates and burning biomass for fuel does not disturb the natural cycle of carbon, nor does it lead to the buildup of toxic waste in the body or in the environment. When plants are converted directly into energy, their stored carbon is simply returned to the atmosphere, and the balance between carbon dioxide and oxygen remains fairly stable.

Along with the surface cycle of carbon is another deeper cycle. Millions of years ago, decaying plants started to accumulate and gradually sink below the earth's surface, eventually taking the form of a thick, dark liquid. Compared to plants at the surface of the earth, this liquid form of carbon—petroleum—exists deep within the earth and is yang or concentrated. And deep within the earth over millions of years, some of these decaying plants became even more yang—fossilized and solid—taking the form of coal. Rather than limiting our involvement in the carbon cycle to its surface aspects, as our ancestors did for thousands of years, modern civilization has dug deep into the earth, brought these concentrated forms of carbon up to the surface, and burnt them for energy.

Fossil fuels are created by time, pressure, and heat, all of which are yang factors. When we burn them, their concentrated energy is suddenly released. Burning these concentrated forms of carbon creates a great deal of waste. Because oil and coal are yang, they contain substances that are resistant to heat and don't burn well. These substances are discharged into the atmosphere, causing pollution. The carbon in fossil fuels was buried long ago. Burning them increases the amount of carbon dioxide in the atmosphere. It also creates a variety of trace gases such as carbon monoxide, methane, sulfur dioxide, nitric oxide, and others that contribute to acid rain, smog, decreased visibility, corrosion, and the greenhouse effect. In addition to the 5 billion tons of carbon dioxide produced each year by burning fossil fuels, the clearing and burning of tropical rain forests (primarily for raising cattle) adds between 0.6 billion and 2.6 billion tons of carbon dioxide to the atmosphere, together with trace gases such as those mentioned above.

In *State of the World*, Sandra Postel of the Worldwatch Institute describes the increase in atmospheric carbon that has resulted from these activities:

> Since 1860, the combustion of fossil fuels has released some 185 billion tons of carbon into the atmosphere. Annual emissions rose from an estimated 93 million tons in 1860 to about 5 billion tons at present, a fifty-three-fold increase. The bulk of these emissions occurred since 1950 as the rapid rise in oil use added substantially to carbon releases from coal.

On the whole, the atmosphere is becoming more yang— thick and dense—as a result of the buildup of carbon dioxide, trace gases, metals, and other forms of pollution. The burning of fossil fuels, smelting, incineration, and other high temperature processes have increased the concentration of yang elements in the environment. For example, worldwide lead emissions now total about 2 million tons per year, largely as the result of using lead in gasoline. That is more than 300 times greater than the amount of lead entering the environment from natural sources.

The atmosphere should be yin—light and clear—in order to balance the hard, compact structure of the earth. The two main components of the atmosphere, nitrogen and oxygen, are yin gases. Animals are yang, and when the atmosphere is yin, it nourishes and makes balance with them. The increasing level of air pollution poses a direct threat to human health as well as to the environment. According to Sandra Postel:

> The same fossil fuel pollutants damaging forests and crops also harm people. Metals released into the environment have become a growing cause for concern. Most recently, the proliferation of synthetic chemicals applied to crops, dispersed

41

into the air, and disposed of on land has added a new dimension to environmental health risks.

The U.S. Office of Technology Assessment estimates that 50,000 premature deaths in the United States may be due to air pollution, especially the combination of sulfates and particulates in the atmosphere. The damage caused by air pollution is not limited to human beings, but affects all forms of life. As Chief Seattle said, "the beast, the tree, the man—all share the same breath." Modern civilization, in its rush to industrialize and adopt a diet centered on animal food, has ignored Chief Seattle's warning to keep the air unspoiled and pure. If the pollution of the atmosphere is not reversed, not only will future generations be denied the privilege of tasting "wind that is sweetened by the meadow's flowers," but their health and possibly their survival will be threatened.

Global Warming

Although carbon dioxide makes up only about .03 percent of the molecules that comprise the earth's atmosphere, or about 335 parts per million, it plays a pivotal role in regulating global temperature. Many scientists believe that the increasing levels of carbon dioxide and other trace gases in the atmosphere is causing the planet to become warmer. When heat from the sun strikes the earth, some of it is absorbed and the rest is reflected back into space. Proponents of global warming believe that carbon dioxide and other greenhouse gases trap heat in the way that glass prevents heat from escaping from a greenhouse. Hence the name "greenhouse effect."

The atmosphere acts as a screen that allows various types of radiation to pass through. For millions of years, the atmosphere efficiently absorbed enough heat to keep temperatures within the moderate range needed for the development of life. However, increasing concentrations of carbon dioxide in the atmosphere mean that the mesh of the screen is becoming tight and yang. Light from the sun has a shorter wavelength and can pass through the atmospheric screen. However, heat radiated by the earth's surface takes the form of infrared radiation which has a longer wavelength. These waves are dense and yang, and cannot pass so easily through the narrowing mesh of the atmosphere. As a result, the atmosphere traps heat rather than releasing it. It is this retention of heat that may be causing a rise in average global temperatures.

In *State of the World*, Lester Brown and Sandra Postel describe research documenting the rise in average temperatures throughout the world:

> In late July 1986, a team of scientists studying the effect of rising atmospheric levels of carbon dioxide (CO_2) and other "greenhouse gases" published evidence that the predicted global warming has begun. Meteorologists at the University of East Anglia in the United Kingdom constructed a comprehensive global temperature series for the last 134 years. Their conclusion: "The data show a long time scale warming trend, with the three warmest years being 1980, 1981 and 1983, and five of nine warmest years in the entire 134-year record occurring after 1978." Three months later, a U.S. Geological Survey team reported that the frozen earth beneath the Arctic tundra in Alaska had warmed 4-7 degrees Fahrenheit (2.2-3.9 degrees Celsius) over the last century, providing further evidence that a CO_2-induced warming was under way.

Studies of Antarctic ice also reveal that in the past, periods of global warming (such as those occurring between ice ages) were accompanied by a rise in the concentration of carbon dioxide in the atmosphere. Cooling periods were accompanied by a drop in the concentration of carbon dioxide. Researchers believe that a doubling of atmospheric carbon dioxide over pre-industrial levels will produce a rise in average temperatures by between 1.5 and 4.5 degrees Celsius. If present trends continue, a doubling of atmospheric carbon dioxide is predicted to occur around the middle of the next cen-

43

tury.

Aside from producing profound changes in the earth's climatic and weather patterns, a rise in the average global temperature by as little as 3 degrees Celsius could cause the polar ice to melt. If that were to happen, the ocean could rise by up to five meters, submerging New York, Boston, San Francisco and other coastal cities. The Great Lakes could spill over their banks, flooding cities such as Chicago and Toronto, and forming a huge inland sea in the middle of North America. Parts of Japan and England would also be under water, and the coastline of Europe would change drastically. Melting of the polar ice could also alter the rotation of the earth, leading to a sudden shift in the earth's polar axis that would cause immediate worldwide devastation.

Sir Crispin Tickell, a British environmentalist, commented on civilization's vulnerability to climatic change in a speech to the Royal Society in London:

> A heavy concentration of people is at present in low-lying coastal areas along the world's great river systems. Nearly one third of humanity lives within sixty kilometers of a coastline. A rise in mean sea level of only twenty-five centimeters would have substantial effects—a problem of an order of magnitude which no one has ever had to face.

Modern civilization's interference with the natural carbon cycle mirrors its inefficient use of carbon in the food chain. The modern diet is a primary contributor—both directly and indirectly—to the buildup of carbon dioxide and other greenhouse gases in the atmosphere. Instead of eating plant foods directly, grains and beans are used to feed livestock. The average American consumes 179 pounds of red meat and poultry every year. Thus cows, pigs, and chickens are being used as middlemen between human beings and the vegetable kingdom, even though the human digestive system is ideally suited to plant foods.

Converting plant food to animal food wastes energy and

natural resources and is harmful to human health. At present, nearly 40 percent of the world's grain is fed to livestock. Thirty-three percent of all the raw materials consumed by the United States is used solely for the production of meat, dairy, and eggs. Growing grains and vegetables uses 95 percent less raw materials as compared with meat production. In order to meet the American demand for meat, 190 gallons of water is required each day for each person in the United States. It takes 2,500 gallons of water to produce a 1 pound steak, and 100 gallons to produce one pat of butter. Only 25 gallons are required to produce a pound of wheat. Livestock production requires more than half of all the water used in the United States.

According to David Pimental, a researcher at Cornell University, corn or wheat return 22 times more protein per calorie of fossil fuel than beef produced on the modern feedlot. Soybeans are 40 times more energy-efficient than modern beef. It takes only a little more than a barrel of oil to produce one ton of grain. If the entire world were to adopt a modern meat-centered diet, all the world's known reserves of oil would be depleted within thirteen years.

Increasing dependence on animal foods and refined carbohydrates in the diet is equivalent to increasing dependence on fossil fuels. Rising consumption of meat and sugar during the 20th century parallels the increasing concentration of carbon dioxide in the atmosphere. In a 1978 study, researcher Maurice Green reported that the per capita use of energy for modern food processing and production comes to the equivalent of 375.4 gallons of oil per year, or about 1 gallon of gasoline a day. This includes the energy used in the manufacture of heavy farm equipment, chemical fertilizers and pesticides, and in processing and refining. The major users of fossil fuels are the meat and meat products industry and the sugar industry. These are followed by the beverage and soft drink industry.

The modern food system also disrupts the nitrogen cycle. The widespread use of nitrogen-based fertilizers adds substantial quantities of nitrous oxide to the atmosphere. Nitrous oxide is a greenhouse gas, and is also produced by the con-

Rise in Carbon Dioxide in Atmosphere Parallels Rise of Meat and Sugar Consumption

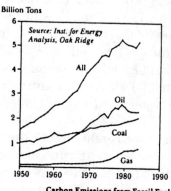

Carbon Emissions from Fossil Fuel
Combustion Worldwide, 1950-84

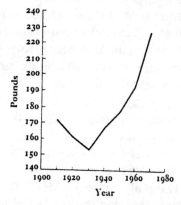

Source: USDA/ERS, 1975

Per capita consumption of
meat, poultry and fish

Source: HSPA Manual, 1972

Per capita annual refined sugar consumption

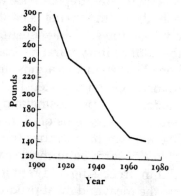

Source: USDA/ERS, 1975

Per capita cereal products
consumption

centration of animal wastes in modern feedlots. The US cattle population produces 158 million tons of animal waste each year. Once released, nitrous oxide may remain in the atmosphere for a century or more. By 2030, the concentration of nitrous oxide in the atmosphere could increase global warming by 20 percent above the level predicted to occur because of carbon dioxide.

A meat-centered diet contributes not only to the buildup of greenhouse gases, but to the direct pollution of the atmosphere. Researchers from Caltech reported in 1991 that cooking meat contributes to air pollution by releasing hydrocarbons, furans, steroids, and pesticide residues. In Los Angeles, long noted for its smog, barbecued beef was the greatest source of fine organic particles in the atmosphere, substantially exceeding fireplaces, gasoline- and diesel-powered vehicles, dust from road paving, forest fires, organic chemical processing, metallurgical processing, jet aircraft, and cigarettes.

To reduce global warming, in 1991 the Worldwatch Institute called for curtailing meat and poultry production. Overgrazing, deforestation, water pollution, and methane emissions from raising livestock are a principal cause of global warming, the agency reported. Flatulence by domestic animals alone accounts for 3 percent of worldwide methane production, another carbon compound that acts as a greenhouse gas. Unrefined complex carbohydrate foods, such as whole grains, beans, fresh local vegetables, and sea-vegetables require far less energy to produce and transport. A large-scale shift to a diet based on unrefined complex carbohydrates would substantially reduce the amount of energy used by each person, and contribute to a reduction of carbon dioxide and other greenhouse gases in the atmosphere.

In order to slow the expected rise in global temperatures, scientists estimate that fossil fuel emissions would have to be cut by about 60 percent. Unfortunately, however, as the modern diet and way of life spread around the globe, economists predict that these emissions will actually double over the next forty years. If these forecasts are accurate, nothing less than a global revolution in consciousness, followed by a shift in diet and lifestyle, will be sufficient to reverse this trend.

Destruction of the Rain Forest

Nowhere are the repercussions of the modern diet more apparent than in the wholesale destruction of the tropical rain forests. If we view the earth from a distance, we see that centripetal or contracting force (yang) is stronger at the poles, and centrifugal or expanding energy (yin) is more powerful at the equator. As a result the earth is flatter at the poles and bulges at the equator. This difference creates two completely opposite types of ecology on the earth, which we can refer to as yin ecology and yang ecology. Yin ecology is prevalent in the tropical regions, while yang ecology is found as you move north or south toward the poles.

The predominance of yin energy at the equator creates lush and expanded forms of plant life, while yang energy creates contracted vegetation. As you move away from the equator into the temperate zones, vegetation becomes progressively more contracted, until it disappears entirely in the polar regions. As you move toward the equator, water exists in the yin forms of liquid and water vapor (except at very high altitudes); while at the poles it assumes the yang, solid form of ice.

Planetary Energies

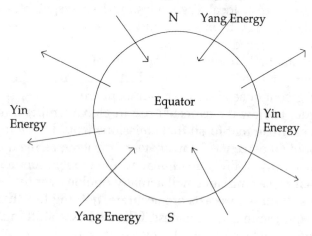

48

The composition of water also changes. Water in the temperate zones contains a higher concentration of yang minerals, while water in the tropical zones contains a greater proportion of living organisms, including bacteria, which are yin in comparison to minerals. The ocean water of the Far North contains a higher proportion of salt than the ocean water at the equator.

Tropical rain forests are a product of the strong centrifugal force at the equator. Rain forests are found in a belt that stretches around the equator, including the Amazon jungle in Brazil, and the jungles of West Africa, Malaysia, and New Guinea. Rain forests have a very yin, fragile ecology, and among other things, are storehouses for a wide range of plant and animal life.

Strong yin energy at the equator creates the wide range of biodiversity found in the rain forest. Biodiversity, or the proliferation of plant and animal species, becomes less as you move toward the poles. For example, there might be only several species of beetles in northern Canada, while in a tropical rain forest there are thousands. Tropical forests cover less than 6 percent of the earth's surface, an area about the size of the contiguous United States, yet contain more than 50 percent of the planet's species. Some experts claim that as many as 90 percent of all living species survive nowhere else but in the tropical rain forest.

Writing in *National Geographic,* Harvard biologist Edward O. Wilson described the diversity of life in the rain forest:

> In just one 25-acre tract in Malaysia, Peter Ashton of Harvard University found 750 species of trees. In another record-breaking survey, Alwyn Gentry of the Missouri Botanical Garden identified 283 tree species in only 2.5 acres near Iquitos, Peru. By contrast, about 700 species make up the entire native tree flora of the United States and Canada. Animal diversity is equally mind-boggling. From a single tree in Amazonia, I identified 43 ant species, approximately the same number as occur in all the British Isles.

As we move toward the equator, strong yin energy causes the range of colors in the natural world to increase. The birds, insects, animals, and plants in the tropical forest come in a stunning variety of colors, as do the fish in tropical oceans. The range of colors in the biological world becomes narrower as we move toward the poles. Animals in the temperate zones, for example, come in fewer and more subdued colors, and have no color at all when we reach the polar regions. Penguins, polar bears, and Arctic seals are thus black and white.

Yin and Yang Ecology

Yin Ecology	Yang Ecology
Created by centrifugal energy	Created by centripetal energy
Found in tropical areas	Found in temperate and polar regions
Produces lush, expanded vegetation	Produces sparse and contracted vegetation
Produces ocean water with more salt	Produces ocean water with less salt
Contains more biodiversity and colorful life	Contains less biodiversity and less colorful life
Causes a greater proportion of soil nutrients to be held above	Causes a greater proportion of soil nutrients to be held below the ground
Produces species with less adaptability	Produces species with wide adaptability
Generates oxygen and absorbs carbon dioxide	Generates carbon dioxide and absorbs oxygen

Conversely, the adaptability of species becomes less as we move toward the equator. The plants and animals in the rain forest are highly specialized and able to live only within a narrow range of environmental conditions, in contrast to the wide adaptability of species in the temperate zones.

The Indians of South America refer to the rain forest as the lungs of the planet. As we saw above, oxygen is yin and carbon dioxide yang. Because yin energy is stronger at the equator, the tropical forests are something like huge processing plants that manufacture oxygen. They also absorb a tremendous amount of carbon dioxide.

However, modern civilization has launched all-out war on this precious natural resource. An area of the earth's rain forests the size of a football field is now destroyed every second. Cattle ranching is the leading cause of tropical deforestation. Al Gore describes the tragic destruction of the tropical rain forests in *Earth in the Balance*:

> As it happens, some of the most disturbing images of environmental destruction can be found exactly halfway between the North and South poles—precisely at the equator in Brazil—where billowing clouds of smoke regularly blacken the sky above the immense but now threatened Amazon rain forest. Acre by acre, the rain forest is being burned to create fast pasture for fast-food beef, with more than one Tennessee's worth of rain forest being slashed and burned each year.

Because the tropical ecology is so yin and fragile, 95 percent of the soil nutrients in the rain forest exist above the ground in the form of plant life. More than half of the plant and animal species also live high above the ground in the rain forest canopy, the thick upper foliage where more than 90 percent of photosynthesis takes place. In the yang, temperate deciduous forests, 95 percent of the nutrients are found in the soils and 5 percent are found in the forest itself. Northern forests have stronger powers of regeneration than the fragile forests of the tropics.

When developers level a section of the rain forest with chain saws and bulldozers, they remove 95 percent of the nutrient base, leaving a thin layer of nutrients below the soil. Then, they plant grass and bring in cattle to graze. But, because the soil is so thin, the cattle rapidly exhaust it. When the land is no longer fertile, they move to another section of the forest and again destroy the native plant and animal species, plant grass, and bring in cattle. Then when the soil in that section is depleted, they move to another part of the forest and repeat the same process.

Because vegetation is yin, forests store water. The forests of the earth store more water than all of the earth's lakes. When rain forests are destroyed, rainfall declines and the region becomes drier. In Ethiopia, for example, the amount of forested land has decreased from 40 percent to 1 percent in the last forty years. The amount of rainfall has also decreased, so that the country is becoming a dry wasteland, with repeated droughts and famine. Destruction of the Amazon rain forest could disrupt the hydrological cycle and produce a similar reaction throughout Central and South America.

Before modern civilization, there were about six million square miles of tropical rain forests on the earth. The amount of rain forest has now been reduced by half, to about three million square miles. At the current rate of destruction, virtually all of the tropical rain forests will vanish by the middle of the next century. Humanity will lose an invaluable natural resource, with unfathomable consequences.

According to scientists at the National Academy of Sciences Forum on Biodiversity held in 1986, the magnitude of species extinction caused by destruction of the rain forests may equal that which led to extinction of the dinosaurs sixty million years ago. Species are now vanishing one thousand times faster than at any time since the disappearance of the dinosaurs. The destruction of so many species in such a short time would represent an irreparable tear in the delicate fabric of life.

As Chief Seattle said nearly a century and a-half ago, "Man did not weave the web of life; he is merely a strand in it. Whatever he does to the web, he does to himself." Those of us in the modern world would be wise to heed Chief Seattle's warning. If we are indeed one with the spiral of life, the total destruction of the tropical rain forests and the disappearance of an unaccountable number of plant and animal species will not fail to have consequences for our own species. Destruction of the rain forest and the species it contains may be the most urgent environmental issue of our time.

Ozone Depletion

Surrounding the earth, high in the stratosphere, between 10 and 30 miles up, is a very thin layer of gas known as ozone. Ozone (O_3) is made up of three atoms of oxygen. Oxygen commonly exists in the molecular form (O_2) in which two atoms of oxygen are combined. The understanding of yin and yang can help us understand how ozone is formed and why the fragile layer of ozone at the periphery of the atmosphere is so important to life on earth.

Overall, the sun is yang: bright, hot, and intense. However, sunlight polarizes into yin and yang wavelengths. The yin, shortwave form of solar radiation is called ultraviolet. The yang, long wave form is called infrared. Visible light is in between these two poles. Ozone is formed when strong yin ultraviolet radiation strikes oxygen molecules high in the stratosphere. As we saw earlier, oxygen is a yin element. Ultraviolet light causes oxygen molecules to become yang; splitting them into two highly energetic atoms of oxygen $(O_2 \rightarrow O + O)$. These highly energetic atoms are attracted to and readily combine with less energetic oxygen molecules, forming a molecule of ozone $(O + O_2 \rightarrow O_3)$. The addition of an atom of oxygen to the oxygen molecule makes ozone more concentrated or yang than molecular oxygen.

Ozone also occurs at ground level as a part of what is known as photochemical smog. Because it is more concentrated than normal oxygen, it produces a variety of unpleasant effects on plants and animals. In humans, it causes eye irritation and impaired lung function. It also damages trees and crops.

When ultraviolet rays strike the ozone layer in the stratosphere, they react in a different way than infrared rays do. As we saw, ozone is concentrated or yang, and ultraviolet light is yin. Since opposites attract, most of the ultraviolet radiation from the sun is absorbed by the ozone, while infrared radiation—which is yang—is repelled and allowed to pass through. Yin ultraviolet radiation can be damaging to biological life. Fortunately, strongly yin ultraviolet rays are filtered out by ozone. Because of the ozone layer, solar radiation has had a beneficial influence that is conducive to life.

Sun, Earth, and Ozone Layer

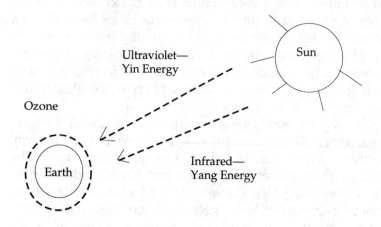

The balance of the upper atmosphere has existed for billions of years. Because of the protection afforded by the ozone shield, life was able to develop and flourish. However, in the 20th century, the fragile balance of the outer atmosphere has been disturbed. In the 1920s, chemists first synthesized chemicals known as chlorofluorocarbons, or CFCs. They are made up of chlorine, flourine, and carbon atoms. These chemicals do not combine easily with other substances, and are used as coolants in refrigerators and propellant gases for spray cans. They are also are used as insulators in plastic-foam materials such as Styrofoam. By 1987, there were an estimated 2.1 billion pounds of CFCs in use throughout the world. There is now twice as much chlorine in the stratosphere as there would be naturally, largely because of CFC emissions.

CFCs damage the environment in two ways: a molecule of CFC is 20,000 times more efficient than a molecule of carbon dioxide at trapping heat. CFCs thus contribute to global warming. Secondly, CFCs gradually migrate up to the outer reaches of the stratosphere. Ultraviolet radiation high above the earth causes CFC molecules to break up and release energized chlorine atoms that destroy ozone. Energized chlorine atoms are attracted to ozone molecules. They fuse with less energetic oxygen atoms that are locked in ozone molecules. The result is the formation of chlorine monoxide and molecular oxygen: $(Cl + O_3 \rightarrow ClO + O_2)$.

Chlorine monoxide then reacts with an oxygen atom formed when ultraviolet light splits another ozone molecule. The two oxygen atoms combine and the chlorine is liberated: $(ClO + O \rightarrow Cl + O_2)$. The chlorine atom is again attracted to ozone, thus beginning the cycle again. One atom of chlorine destroys many molecules of ozone.

The relationship between CFCs and destruction of the ozone layer was discovered in the 1970s. In 1985, researchers found a hole in the ozone layer over Antarctica. The Antarctic ozone hole is now estimated to cover an area three times larger than the contiguous United States. In 1991, the U.S. Environmental Protection Agency reported that the ozone has also been depleted over the earth's mid-latitudes, including the United States. The ozone shield above the United States may be at its thinnest in summer when the risk of ultraviolet radiation is greatest.

In spite of recent reductions in the amount of CFC emissions, scientists believe that the ozone layer may lose 5 to 7 percent of its effectiveness over the next twenty years, due to the fact that the CFCs already released in the environment will take another fifteen to twenty years to reach the stratosphere. According to some estimates, there will be 17 percent less ozone over North America in 2010 than there was in the 1960s. CFCs remain in the atmosphere for up to fifty years after being released.

As a result of ozone depletion, a larger amount of ultraviolet radiation will reach the earth, with potentially harmful effects for plant and animal life. For every 1 percent decrease in ozone, there is a 2 percent increase in the amount of ultraviolet radiation reaching the planet. The human immune system is affected by solar radiation, in addition to being affected by diet and emotions. A variety of white blood cells, or lymphocytes, are involved in the body's immune response. One category of cells, known as T-cells, regulate the immune response either by activating or shutting it off. T-cells come in yin and yang varieties. Yang T-helper cells activate the immune response. T-suppressor cells are yin and turn it off.

Because they are yin, ultraviolet rays inhibit T-helper cells and activate T-suppressor cells, thus diminishing natural immunity. By letting more ultraviolet rays through, ozone depletion could weaken people's immune function, and, when coupled with the immune-depleting effects of the modern diet, lead to increases in melanoma and other forms of skin cancer, AIDS, and infectious diseases.

Erosion of the ozone shield also affects phytoplankton, the tiny, single-cell plants that form the base of the food chain in the oceans. Researchers estimate that the ozone hole over the Antarctic has doubled the intensity of springtime ultraviolet rays reaching that part of the world, and have found a corresponding decline in the growth of phytoplankton. These microscopic organisms are a major source of nutrition for other forms of marine life, and their loss could have a disastrous effect on the food chain as a whole.

Moreover, scientists have discovered that large pieces of the Antarctic ozone hole break off each year around November and float northward. Cataracts and skin cancer have thus become increasingly common in areas of the Southern Hemisphere, while in Patagonia, blind rabbits and salmon have recently been captured by hunters and fishermen.

Diet and Ozone Depletion

Depletion of the ozone layer can be traced to the modern diet. CFCs are used as coolants in refrigerators. The need for refrigeration is increased by the modern reliance on animal foods. The primary foods in the modern diet, eggs, milk, meat, butter, cheese, chicken, and other animal products, require constant refrigeration; otherwise, they rapidly decompose into toxic bacteria and compounds such as ammonia. At the same time, constant refrigeration is required to freeze or chill foods of the opposite extreme, such as ice cream, soft drinks, and frozen orange juice, that are taken to balance the high consumption of animal food.

Air conditioners are another source of CFCs. Automobile air conditioners may be responsible for up to 25 percent of all CFCs entering the atmosphere. Over-reliance on air conditioning is related to the modern diet. A diet high in meat, eggs, chicken, cheese, and other animal foods causes the body to retain heat. For someone eating plenty of animal fat, being in hot weather can be unbearable, while people who base their diets on whole grains, beans, vegetables, and other plant foods don't find hot weather uncomfortable. Even if they live in the South or in big cities, they can usually get by with less air conditioning than people who eat a lot of animal food.

Even though the United States banned the use of CFC-based aerosol spray cans, other countries are still using them. The CFCs in deodorant sprays have contributed to ozone depletion. The need for deodorants is also related to diet, especially consumption of meat and other animal foods. People who eat grains and vegetables do not produce unpleasant body odor and rarely need deodorant.

Foam products, including those used in fast-food containers, are also a major source of CFCs. They account for approximately 28 percent of all the CFCs now entering the atmosphere, according to Sarah Clark of the Environmental Defense Fund. As Al Gore stated in *Newsweek*, "Much of what reaches the atmosphere is not coming from industrial sources. It's things like sloppy handling of hamburger containers." A large-scale shift to a grain- and vegetable-based diet, with emphasis on home cooking, would considerably reduce the use of these products.

The New Ecology

The modern diet is closely tied to each of the environmental problems described above. As the diet of modern civilization has become increasingly out-of-balance, so has civilization's relationship with the environment. In a survey of organizations and individuals in the fields of nutrition and ecology, including Frances Moore Lappé, author of *Diet for a Small Planet*; David Pimental of Cornell University's College of Agriculture; John Robbins, founder of Earthsave and author of *Diet for a New America*; and Robin Hur, an Oregon-based researcher, *Vegetarian Times* summarized findings showing that a plant-based diet could contribute to a healthier planet:

- More than 50 percent of tropical rain forest destruction (216,000 acres per day) is linked with livestock production.
- An average of 55 square feet of forest is destroyed for every hamburger produced from cattle raised in former Central American rain forests.
- The current rate of species extinction from loss of tropical rain forests and related habitats is 1,000 per year.
- One acre of trees is saved each year by by each person who switches to a plant-based diet.
- The average amount of water required daily for a vegetarian who eats dairy food and eggs is about 1,200 gallons, about 25 percent the amount for someone eating the standard American diet. The amount of water required for a person on a dairy-free, plant-based diet is 300 gallons.
- About 85 percent of the topsoil loss in the United States is directly connected with livestock production.
- A reduction in meat consumption by only 10 percent would free enough grain in the United States to feed an estimated 60 million people

worldwide.
  • More than 50 percent of the water pollution in the United States is associated with animal food production and chemical farming.
  • Imported oil could be cut by 60 percent if the nation switched to a plant-based diet.

The relationship between what we eat and the health of the environment is becoming increasingly clear. Switching to a macrobiotic diet based on whole grains and vegetables benefits not only our personal health and well being, but the health and well being of the planet. Macrobiotics stresses the importance of eating locally-grown foods in season, and relying on foods in their natural, unprocessed state. Both of these recommendations reduce the use of energy and fossil fuels. Macrobiotics also recommends natural and organic farming methods as well as home cooking.

According to the National Academy of Sciences report, *Alternative Agriculture*, the chemicals used in modern agriculture have been associated with causing cancer, behavioral effects, altered immune system function, and allergic reactions. Insecticides accounting for 30 percent, herbicides accounting for 50 percent, and fungicides accounting for 90 percent of all agricultural use have been found to cause tumors in laboratory animals. A shift toward organic farming would reduce or eliminate these hazards to personal and environmental health.

In the human body, a steady diet of animal foods causes saturated fat and cholesterol to accumulate in the blood, eventually clogging the arteries and blood vessels. If the accumulation of excess continues unchecked, it can lead to collapse of the body due to heart attack or stroke, or to accumulation of waste products and other toxins in the organs leading to cancer.

On a planetary level, the modern diet and way of life have contributed to the buildup of toxins in the environment that threatens the earth's ecosystem. And just as a diet based on animal protein and fat leads to an acidic blood condition, the burning of carbon compounds, especially high-sulfur coal, has caused the atmosphere to become acidic. Acid rain has already destroyed crops and forests and made our soils and waterways toxic, in the same way that an over-acid blood condition causes a loss of minerals in the body and damages cells.

As we move up the food chain from plants to animals, yang, or contracting energy, becomes stronger. Animals represent the condensation of a great deal of plant food. Strong yang energy causes the toxic chemicals used in modern agriculture to accumulate in animal tissues to a far greater degree than they do in plants. These toxins concentrate especially in fat cells. According to John Robbins, 95 to 99 percent of all pesticides and other toxic residues in the American diet come from meat, dairy products, eggs, and other animal foods. Plant foods contain relatively low concentrations of chemical residues. We can substantially reduce the buildup of these toxins in our bodies and in the environment by eating whole grains, beans, fresh local vegetables, and other foods that are lower on the food chain, and by selecting organically grown foods whenever possible.

By eating energy-efficient foods in harmony with climate and season, produced by organic methods, we support a system of farming and food production that will preserve the soil, water, and air for a countless number of future generations. A balanced natural foods diet, respect for nature, and ecological living underlie the macrobiotic way of life and are a direct solution to the environmental crisis. Eating whole grains, beans, fresh local vegetables, and other whole natural foods is the most important step that each of us can take to restore not only our personal health, but the health of the environment.

Part Three
Healing Planet Earth

"No illness which can be treated by diet should be treated by any other means."—Maimonides

Early in the 20th century, F.H. King, a professor of agricultural science at the University of Wisconsin, journeyed to Asia to study traditional farming practices. He found that people in China, Korea, and Japan were practicing a form of sustainable agriculture that had, over thousands of years, provided food for millions of people. His travels were chronicled in *Farmers of Forty Centuries*, published in 1911. Professor King made two discoveries that may help explain the success of Oriental farming methods. His discoveries also have important implications for the environmental crisis.

His first discovery, made more than half a century before publication of *Diet for a Small Planet*, has to do with the economy of a diet based on whole grains and vegetables:

> It is true that they are vegetarians to a far higher degree than are most western nations, and the high maintenance efficiency of the agriculture of China, Korea and Japan is in great measure rendered possible by the adoption of a diet so largely vegetarian. Hopkins, in his *Soil Fertility and Permanent Agriculture*, makes this pointed statement of fact: "1000 bushels of grain has at least five

times as much food value and will support five times as many people as will the meat or milk that can be made from it."

The second observation has to do with the traditional practice of recycling and soil maintenance:

> For centuries, all cultivated lands, including adjacent hill and mountain sides, the canals, streams and the sea have been made to contribute what they could toward the fertilization of cultivated fields. In China, in Korea, and in Japan all but the inaccessible portions of their vast extent of mountain and hill lands have long been taxed to their full capacity for fuel, lumber and herbage for green manure and compost material; and the ash of practically all of the fuel and of all the lumber used at home finds its way ultimately to the fields as fertilizer.

Professor King believed that people in the West could learn valuable lessons from the rice, millet, and vegetable farmers of the Orient. Unfortunately, his study appeared at the dawn of mechanized, chemical farming, and at a time when consumption of animal food was beginning to increase, so that his suggestions were not taken seriously. However, given the negative environmental and health effects of the modern meat-centered diet and chemical farming, it is now time to revisit Professor King's discoveries.

For thousands of years, people in the Orient (and in traditional Western cultures) based their diet and agriculture on whole cereal grains, beans, and fresh local vegetables. Animal food was an occasional supplement, more in the West than in the East, and people ate the foods that grew in their local area. Moreover, having been schooled in the understanding of yin and yang, the universal principles of harmony and balance, people in Oriental countries practiced a self-sustaining form of agriculture based on balancing what they took from the earth (yin) with what they returned to it (yang). Traditional farmers oriented their cycles of planting, cultivation, and harvest with the eternal cycles of nature. They practiced strict organic farming and understood the importance of keeping the soil in a healthy natural state. It was because of these practices that the soil was consistently able to produce food for over 4,000 years.

These time-tested practices not only hold the key to a sustainable agriculture, but to a sustainable future. Changing to a grain-based diet and practicing sustainable organic farming are the first steps toward solving the environmental crisis as well as problems of personal health. Modern environmental and health problems are interrelated and can be traced to society's failure to observe these simple practices.

Finding a solution to the environmental crisis begins with individuals. Concern for the environment is meaningless if it is not backed by action. Daily life is the proving ground for our environmental beliefs. True environmentalism is based on deeds, and not only on words. Individual actions reverberate throughout society and produce either a positive or negative impact on the environment.

Responsible consumption is the first step toward restoring harmony with the environment. Responsible consumption encourages responsible production. Each of us can choose what to consume and what not to consume. It is also the first step in restoring personal health. Personal health and planetary health are one. Food is our primary link with the environment, the bridge between our internal and external worlds. A diet that benefits our health benefits the environment. A diet that is harmful for personal health also harms the environment.

Disruption of the planetary environment during the 20th century corresponds to the shift from humanity's traditional diet, based around centrally-balanced foods such as whole grains, beans, fresh local vegetables, and other complex carbohydrate-foods, to the modern diet based on extremes such as meat, eggs, chicken, dairy and other animal products, as well as refined sugar, processed flour, and chemically-produced foods. The decline of environmental health corresponds to the rise of chronic illness during the same period.

Central to the new ecology is the awareness that a healthy environment begins with our own health. Each of us can take responsibility not only for our own health, but ultimately for the health and well being of our planet.

Changing to a diet of whole grains and vegetables produces immediate and practical benefits both for our personal health and the environment. Planetary ecology begins with your local organic grower, continues at the natural food store in your neighborhood, and is brought to fruition at home in your kitchen. There is no better way to put into practice Buckminster Fuller's advice to think globally but act locally. What could be more local than your own body and the food you put into it every day?

There are encouraging signs that the relationship between diet, personal health, and the environment is now being taken seriously, especially by young people. In the spring of 1993 I met with director and staff of Friends of the Earth in Washington, D.C. The purpose of our meeting was to discuss the role of a naturally balanced diet in personal and planetary health. During the discussion, one member of the staff stated that changing to a grain-based diet had become the single most common environmentally-motivated action taken by FoE members around the world. In Great Britain, half of the teenage girls have adopted vegetarian diets, largely because of environmental concerns, while in the United States, teenage girls represent the fastest growing group of new vegetarians. At the same time, 84 percent of American students said they would take environmental action if they had more information on what to do. The people who will inherit the 21st century seem to be getting the message about the importance of preserving the environment and about a balanced natural diet. Below are twelve basic steps that can guide you in your transition toward a healthful and ecological diet and lifestyle.

1. Eat Lower on the Food Chain.

As we move up the food chain from plant to animal foods, the amount of energy required to produce, transport, and store foods increases dramatically. Grains, vegetables, beans, sea vegetables, and other plant foods are lower on the food chain and require much less energy to produce. Researchers at Ohio State University compared the amounts of energy required to produce plant and animal foods and discovered that the least energy-efficient plant food was still nearly 10 times as efficient as the most energy-efficient animal food. Eating a plant-based diet reduces the use of fossil fuels and eases the pollution burden entering your body and the environment, including toxic pesticides and synthetic hormones, as well as greenhouse gases such as carbon dioxide, methane, and nitrous oxide.

2. Base Your Diet on Balanced Foods.

Foods, like everything else in our environment, can be classified into yin and yang. Eggs, meat, chicken, hard cheese, and other animal products, together with foods high in sodium, are strongly yang or contractive; while refined sugar, tropical fruits, spices, coffee, chocolate, ice cream, artificial sweeteners, soft drinks, nightshade vegetables, and foods high in potassium are strongly yin or expansive. Centrally-balanced foods have an even balance of yin and yang—or expansive and contractive energies—and include whole grains, beans, fresh local vegetables, sea vegetables, non-stimulant beverages, and non-spicy seasonings and condiments.

Centrally-balanced foods are also the most energy-efficient. Whole organic foods are beneficial for human health. They are the product of self-sustaining agriculture that does not pollute the environment or waste natural resources. On the other hand, extremes of yin or yang are frequently the product of chemically intensive agriculture and modern industry. Producing them utilizes an excessive amount of natural resources and spoils the environment. It takes 78 calories of fossil fuel to produce 1 calorie of protein from beef. Only 2 calories of fossil fuel are needed to obtain 1 calorie of protein from soybeans.

The negative environmental and health effects of the modern meat-centered diet have been well documented.

Yin and Yang Categories of Food

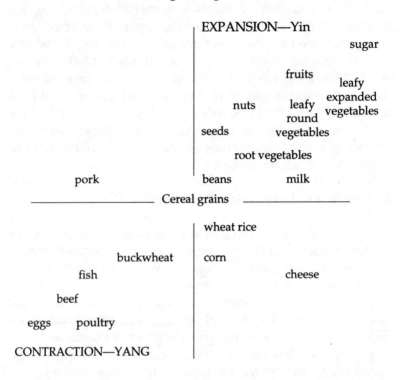

EXPANSION—Yin

sugar

fruits

leafy
expanded
vegetables

nuts   leafy
round
seeds   vegetables

root vegetables

pork   beans   milk

———————— Cereal grains ————————

wheat rice

buckwheat   corn

fish   cheese

beef

eggs   poultry

CONTRACTION—YANG

Because of that, vegetarianism has become a worldwide trend. However, simply avoiding meat and other animal foods is not enough. Extreme yin foods such as refined sugar, chocolate, bananas, pineapples, and other tropical fruits, and processed soft drinks also produce negative health and environmental effects. Sugar production, for example, has historically been a major cause of deforestation. In *Native Roots: How the Indians Enriched America,* Jack Weatherford describes the deforestation of New England and the Caribbean islands in the 1770s:

> New Englanders shipped to the Caribbean the wood from a quarter of a million trees between 1771 and 1773. The sugar mills of the Caribbean boomed in this period, but the Caribbean settlers

had already consumed their own forests to feed the high-temperature fires needed to extract sugar from the cane. The West Indians needed massive amounts of firewood to continue making sugar, and to distill their molasses into rum. The West Indians sold sugar to Europe, but they bought timber from New England to operate these industrial plantations.

Throughout the Third World, where strongly yin crops such as coffee, bananas, sugar, and cocoa are produced, the pattern is the same: land that could be used to produce grains, beans, vegetables, and other staple foods for the local population has been converted to the cultivation of cash crops for export. The appropriation of prime land for cash crops has had devastating consequences for the ecology and economy of these regions. Frances Moore Lappé and Joseph Collins describe how cash cropping has taken over the Caribbean islands in *Food First: Beyond the Myth of Scarcity*:

> Over half of all the arable land in the Caribbean is planted with cash crops for export: sugar cane, cocoa, bananas, tobacco, vegetables, and coffee. In Guadeloupe over 66 percent of the arable land is put to the plow for sugar cane, cocoa, and bananas. In Martinique over 70 percent is planted with sugar cane, cocoa, bananas, and coffee. In Barbados, 77 percent of the arable land grows sugar cane alone.

Most cash crops are grown with chemically intensive farming that pollutes the soil, air, and water. Many of the pesticides banned in the United States are still in use in the developing countries, and are applied intensively to crops grown for export. Moreover, most of the plantations devoted to luxury crops have expropriated the best land for the continuous cultivation of crops, forcing local farmers to retreat onto marginal lands, often on hillsides, that are not suited to intensive farming. These lands are soon ravaged by erosion. In their book, Lappé and Collins offer an insightful contrast between traditional farming and the modern production of export crops:

> In dramatic contrast to cash-cropping monoculture, the traditional and self-provisioning agriculture that it replaces is often quite sound ecologically. It is a long-evolved adaptation to tropical soil and climate. It reflects a sophisticated understanding of the complex rhythms of the local ecosystem. The mixing of crops, sometimes of more than twenty different species, means harvests are staggered and provides maximum security against wholesale losses due to unreasonable weather, pests, or disease. Moreover, mixed cropping provides the soil with year-round protection from the sun and rain.

An ecological diet is based on centrally-balanced foods, and avoids extremes of both yin and yang. As we saw in the first section, the path to health and healing lies in the middle way. Basing your diet on whole grains, beans, and fresh local vegetables is the best way to maintain your health while benefiting the environment.

3. Eat Foods From Your Climatic Zone.

A diet based on animal food is appropriate for the Inuvialuit tribes who inhabit the Arctic region. It is not appropriate for someone living in Houston. The intake of tropical fruits is more appropriate for people in Costa Rica than it is for those in Chicago. Today, however, people in the temperate zones eat a "polar-tropical" diet. They have replaced the whole grains, beans, fresh local vegetables, and other foods appropriate to their region with meat, eggs, cheese, poultry, and other foods suited to cold, polar climates, and with sugar, chocolate, spices, coffee, tropical fruits and vegetables, and other foods suited to equatorial zones.

A tremendous amount of energy is required to maintain

this unnatural dietary pattern. Moreover, as we saw above, the production of such an unbalanced diet has negative consequences for the local ecology. It is far more economical, ecological, and energy-efficient to base your diet around foods that are naturally abundant in your immediate environment or in a climate that is similar to the one in which you are living.

4. Vary Your Diet with the Seasons.

By eating foods that are naturally available in season, we take advantage of the cycles of nature. During the winter, dishes that are strongly seasoned and well cooked help us generate and retain heat. In summer, lightly cooked dishes, including salads, keep us cool. These natural adjustments help us stay in touch with nature and make it easier to adapt to climatic changes without excessive heat in the winter or air conditioning in the summer. Eating fresh seasonal foods reduces the need for refrigeration and other artificial methods of food preservation and storage.

5. Select Organically Grown Foods.

Not only are pesticides harmful to personal health and the environment, they are highly inefficient. In 1945, American farmers lost 3 percent of their corn crop to insects. Today, after widespread use of pesticides, they lose 12 percent. Only 0.1 percent of pesticides sprayed by airplane reach their intended target. The rest damage plants, animals, and people. Moreover, a great deal of fossil fuels are used in the production, transport, and storage of chemical fertilizers, insecticides, herbicides, and other artificial substances used in modern agriculture. When these substances enter the environment, they pollute the air, water, and soil. Nitrous oxide, produced by nitrogen-based fertilizers, is a major greenhouse gas. When you select organically grown foods, you do not contribute to pollution of the environment, the unnecessary use of fossil fuels, or to the buildup of nitrous oxide in the atmosphere.

6. Start a Backyard Garden.

In 1820, 72 percent of Americans were farmers. By 1990, only 2.4 percent were. Modern people have lost their connection with the earth. Growing your own organic vegetables and other foods benefits your health and reduces your reliance on foods that require fossil fuels to package and transport. Many garden vegetables can be left in the soil until they are ready to eat and don't need to be refrigerated. If you don't have space to begin your own garden, look for an organic farm or cooperative in your area. Rather than being thrown away, uneaten food can be recycled as compost in your garden.

7. Eat Foods That Can Be Stored Naturally.

Whole grains, beans, sea vegetables, and other complex carbohydrate foods normally don't require refrigeration or artificial methods of storage or preservation to keep them fresh. They can be kept as is in your pantry or cupboards. On the other hand, meat, eggs, cheese, chicken, and other animal foods rapidly decompose into toxic bacteria and compounds and therefore require artificial preservation. Tropical fruits, vegetables, and other extremely yin foods or drinks also decompose rapidly and thus require refrigeration, canning, or other artificial methods to preserve or keep them fresh.

8. Eat Whole Foods.

Eating foods in their whole form saves energy and makes use of the nutrients that are naturally available. The process whereby brown rice is milled into white rice, or whole wheat flour into white flour, represents an unnecessary waste of energy. The outer coat of cereal grains contains beneficial fiber and other valuable nutrients. When whole grains are refined, these valuable nutrients are lost. The green tops of vegetables such as daikon, carrots, and turnips and the roots of scallions are also a good source of nutrients and can be cooked and eaten rather than discarded.

9. Restore Home Cooking.

A great deal of disposable waste, including paper products, Styrofoam containers, and plastic utensils is generated by restaurants and public eating places. Cooking and eating at home helps reduce the use of the fossil fuels that go into producing these products as well as the buildup of inorganic waste in the environment, including the CFCs contained in plastic foam containers. Moreover, for optimal health, and to minimize electro-pollution, it is better to cook on a gas flame, rather than on the artificial energy of electric stoves or microwave ovens.

10. Make Your Own Snacks and Specialty Foods.

Whenever possible, bake your own whole grain breads, and make foods such as tofu, tempeh, amasake, noodles, pasta, seitan, pickles, and others at home. A great deal of fossil fuels are used in the processing, packaging, and transportation of processed foods. Home processing saves energy. Homemade foods are also fresher and more delicious than those bought at the store.

11. Chew Well.

Thorough chewing allows for the efficient digestion and absorption of foods. When you chew well, you obtain more nutrients from your foods and can get by with a smaller volume of food. Your diet becomes energy-efficient. Both for health and vitality, and to minimize waste, try not to eat for three hours before sleeping, except in unusual circumstances. Also, you might find that your energy levels are higher if you eat a light breakfast or skip breakfast on occasion.

12. Practice an Ecological Lifestyle.

As much as possible, use natural, chemical-free fabrics

and body care products, as well as biodegradable soaps and cleaning materials in your home. Minimize the use of electric devices, in order to conserve energy, for example, by turning off the lights when you are not using a room or watching less television.

Our culture produces a staggering amount of waste. In 1989, Americans used 12 billion pounds of plastic packaging. In the 1990s, this figure is expected to double. To minimize waste, buy your foods in bulk, rather than in individually packaged containers. Sixty-five percent of daily garbage can be attributed to packaging. Recycle paper, glass, and plastic. Americans use 2.5 million plastic bottles every hour, and throw away enough glass jars and bottles each week to fill both 1,350-foot towers at the World Trade Center. The average American college student throws away 500 disposable cups each year. Most of this trash (80 percent) ends up in landfills, yet half of all the trash that is thrown away could be recycled into new products. Unless recycling becomes widespread, mountains of garbage may soon overwhelm the natural landscape.

Recycle leftover food by including it in new dishes rather than throwing it away. In an average school cafeteria, nearly 50 percent of the garbage generated is food waste. The equivalent of about 21 million full shopping bags of food is dumped into American landfills every year. Keep physically active, and rely less on automobiles, elevators, central heating, and air conditioning. Finally, learn to appreciate our planetary environment. Develop gratitude and appreciation for the earth, water, ocean, and air. See your foods as the condensed essence of nature, and offer thanks before and after each meal.

An Ecologically Balanced Diet

The guidelines below are appropriate for those who live in temperate, or four-season climates, such as most of North America, Europe, and the Far East. These guidelines require modification if you live in a tropical or semitropical climate, or a polar or semipolar region. Energy-efficient whole grains, beans, fresh local vegetables, and sea vegetables are the ideal principal foods in all but the most extreme polar climates. The main difference between temperate and tropical diets lies in the varieties of these foods we select and the methods we use to cook them.

Standard Macrobiotic Diet

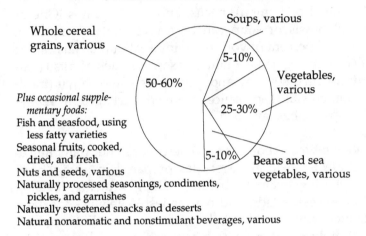

Whole cereal
grains, various

Soups, various

5-10%

50-60%

Vegetables,
various

25-30%

*Plus occasional supple-
mentary foods:*
Fish and seasfood, using
   less fatty varieties
Seasonal fruits, cooked,
   dried, and fresh
Nuts and seeds, various
Naturally processed seasonings, condiments,
   pickles, and garnishes
Naturally sweetened snacks and desserts
Natural nonaromatic and nonstimulant beverages, various

5-10%

Beans and sea
vegetables, various

The guidelines presented below were developed by Michio Kushi, and can be modified to suit an endless variety of circumstances. More detailed food lists and guidelines for practicing a healthful, ecologically balanced diet are presented in the guidebook, *Standard Macrobiotic Diet*, by Michio Kushi, published by One Peaceful World Press.

Foods for Daily Consumption

• **Whole Cereal Grains** Whole grains are the most centrally-balanced foods in terms of yin and yang and are composed largely of energy-efficient complex carbohydrates. They can be the principal food at each meal. They can comprise from 50 to 60 percent of your daily intake by weight. Whole grains include brown rice, sweet brown rice, whole wheat berries, barley, millet, oats, and rye, as well as corn, buckwheat, and other botanically similar plants. From time to time, whole grain products, such as cracked wheat, rolled oats, noodles, pasta, bread, baked goods, seitan (wheat meat), and other unrefined flour products, may be served as a part of your grain intake.

• **Soups** Soups are a hearty and nourishing way to prepare and serve natural foods such as vegetables, sea vegetables (wakame or kombu), beans, and whole grains. One or two small bowls of soup can be served daily, comprising about 5 to 10 percent of your daily intake. Soup broths can be seasoned with vegetable quality seasonings such as miso (naturally fermented soybean and grain purée) and shoyu (traditional, non-chemical soy sauce). Canned, packaged, or ready-made soups are best avoided.

•**Vegetables** About 25 to 30 percent of your daily intake can include fresh local vegetables prepared in a variety of ways, including steaming, boiling, baking, sautéing, pickling (without spices), salads, and marinades. Vegetables for daily use include: green cabbage, kale, broccoli, cauliflower, collards, pumpkin, watercress, Chinese cabbage, bok choy, dandelion, mustard greens, daikon root and greens, scallion, onions, turnips, acorn squash, butternut squash, buttercup squash, burdock, carrots, and other seasonally available varieties. For optimal health, vegetables such as potatoes, sweet potatoes, yams, tomatoes, eggplant, peppers, asparagus, spinach, beets, zucchini, and avocado are best eaten on rare occasions, if at all. Mayonnaise and industrially produced salad dressings are best avoided, as are vegetables brought in from tropical areas.

• **Beans, Bean Products, and Sea Vegetables** About 5 to 10 percent of your daily intake can include cooked beans, bean products, and sea vegetables. Varieties such as azukis, chickpeas, and lentils are good for daily use, as are traditional bean products such as tofu, tempeh, and natto. Sea vegetables are a good source of naturally-available minerals and include wakame, kombu, nori, hiziki, arame, and dulse.

• **Seasoning and Oil** Naturally processed sea salt can be used in seasoning, along with miso, shoyu, umeboshi and brown rice vinegar, fresh grated ginger, and other traditional items. Naturally processed, unrefined vegetable oil is recommended for daily cooking such as sesame seed oil. Kuzu (kudzu) is commonly used for sauces and gravies.

• **Condiments** Condiments include gomashio (roasted sesame salt), roasted sea vegetable powders, umeboshi (pickled plums), tekka root vegetable powder, and others made from whole natural foods.

• **Pickles** A small volume of non-spicy sauerkraut or pickles, made at home or bought at the natural food store, can be eaten daily to aid in digestion of grains and vegetables.

• **Beverages** Spring or well water are recommended for drinking, preparing tea, and for cooking. Bancha twig tea (also known as kukicha) is ideal as a daily beverage, though roasted barley tea, and other grain-based teas or traditional, non-stimulant herbal teas are fine for use.

Occasional Foods

• **Animal Food** A small volume of white-meat fish or seafood may be eaten a few times per week.

• **Seeds and Nuts** Seeds and nuts, lightly roasted and salted with sea salt or seasoned with shoyu, may be enjoyed as occasional snacks.

• **Fruit** Fruit may be eaten several times per week, preferably cooked or naturally dried, as a snack or dessert, provided the fruit grows locally or in a similar climate.

• **Dessert** Occasional desserts, such as cookies, cake, pudding, pie, and other dishes can be made with naturally sweet foods such as apples, fall and winter squashes, azuki beans, chestnuts, or dried fruit, or can be sweetened with grain sweeteners such as rice syrup, barley malt, or amasake.

Foods to Minimize or Avoid

If you live in a temperate climate, avoiding or substantially reducing your intake of the following foods greatly benefits the environment as well as your personal health:

• Meat, animal fat, eggs, poultry, dairy products (including butter, yogurt, ice cream, milk, and cheese), refined sugars, chocolate, molasses, honey, other simple sugars and foods treated with them, and vanilla.

• Tropical or semitropical fruits and fruit juices, soda, artificially flavored drinks and beverages, coffee, colored tea, distilled water, and aromatic or stimulant beverages.

• All artificially colored, preserved, sprayed, chemically treated, or genetically engineered foods. All refined and polished grains, flours, and their derivatives. Mass produced foods including canned, frozen, and irradiated foods. Hot spices, aromatic or stimulant foods, artificial vinegar, and strong alcoholic beverages.

Cooking for Personal and Planetary Health

Cooking is the art of managing our environment. Everyone is advised to learn how to cook by attending cooking classes or studying with an experienced macrobiotic cook. Biodiversity exists within the realm of food as well as within the world of plants and animals. The standard macrobiotic diet includes an incredible range of foods and a wide range of cooking methods can be used to enhance the flavor and appeal of your meals. Macrobiotic cookbooks, such as those listed in the bibliography, can guide you in preparing healthful, delicious, and ecologically balanced meals

Planetary Medicine

Understanding life in terms of energy is the key to healing ourselves and our relationship with the environment. Seeing life in terms of energy widens our perspective considerably. It enables us to perceive the underlying patterns of cause and effect found everywhere in nature. The structures and functions of the human body reflect the universal pattern of energy that comprises all things, including our daily foods. The macrobiotic understanding of yin and yang provides a practical framework for applying the understanding of energy to personal and planetary healing.

In the human body, the inner regions, including the bones, blood, and internal organs, are yang or contracted, while the peripheral regions, including the skin and hair, are yin or expanded. The front of the body is softer and more expanded (yin), while the back is hard and compact (yang). The upper body is yin, while the lower body has stronger yang energy. The right side of the body is strongly charged with yin, upward energy, while on the left side, downward or contracting energy (yang) is stronger. So, for example, the ascending colon moves up the right side, while the descending colon moves down the left. The right hemisphere of the brain generates aesthetic or artistic images, while the left is the source of analytical and rational abilities. Artistic thinking is yin, and is the product of upward energy. Analytical thinking is yang; it is produced primarily by downward, contracting energy. These basic classifications enable us to see how daily foods can be used to nourish and heal our internal condition and our relationship with the environment.

All foods are manifestations of energy. Foods such as meat, chicken, cheese, and eggs are extremely contractive or yang. Sugar, chocolate, ice cream, strong spices, soft drinks, and tropical fruits are extremely expansive or yin. Eating extremes of yin or yang on a regular basis harms the organs and their functions. Extreme foods thus cannot serve as medicine. The word "medicine" means "to walk in the middle." In order to restore the body to a balanced condition, we need to base our diet on centrally balanced whole grains, beans, and fresh local vegetables.

Whole grains are the most balanced among foods. However, each grain has a slightly different quality of energy. Corn, for example, grows in the summer, and is soft, sweet, and juicy. It has a yin quality of energy. Buckwheat, on the other hand, grows in cold, northern regions and is very hard and dry. It rapidly absorbs water, and has strong yang energy. Rice has a different quality of energy than barley; millet is different than wheat. Short grain rice is very different than long grain rice. Certain grains have expansive energies; others are contractive. Because each grain has a different quality of energy, each will affect the body in a different way.

As we saw above, the right side of the body is strongly charged by yin, upward energy. The left side receives a stronger charge of yang, downward energy. Among the cereal grains, which ones nourish the organs on the right side of the body, and which ones nourish those on the left? Which grains help restore balance to the organs in the upper body, and which ones nourish the organs in the lower body? The answer can be found by examining our relationship to the daily cycle of planetary energy.

Day to day, the atmosphere cycles back and forth between upward and downward, or yin and yang energy. Morning is the time when upward energy prevails. Evening and night are the times when downward energy is strongest. In order to maintain optimal health, we need to orient our daily life in harmony with the movement of planetary energy. In other words, we need to be active during the day, and rest at night. If we go against the movement of energy by sleeping during the day and being active at night, we risk losing our health. In the same way, we need to go with the movement of energy in the body by providing each of the organs with foods that have a quality of energy that matches theirs. Healing the organs provides the basis for healing our relationship with the environment. Let us now see how the concept of balancing energy applies to selecting whole grains and other foods to heal and nourish the internal organs.

Five Transformations

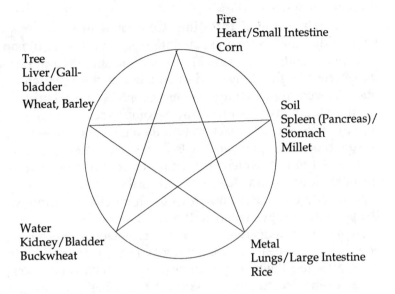

Fire
Heart/Small Intestine
Corn

Tree
Liver/Gall-
bladder
Wheat, Barley

Soil
Spleen (Pancreas)/
Stomach
Millet

Water
Kidney/Bladder
Buckwheat

Metal
Lungs/Large Intestine
Rice

Liver and Gallbladder The liver and gallbladder are located on the right side of the body under the rib cage. Oriental philosopher-healers referred to the upward energy that nourishes these organs as *tree energy*. The name tree energy describes growth in an upward direction, as well as movement that branches outward. The liver and gallbladder comprise a complementary pair of organs—the liver has a yang, solid and compact structure, while the gallbladder has a yin, hollow and expanded form. However, even though they have opposite structures, both are nourished by the upward energy flowing through the right side of the body.

Among the grains, barley has a light, expansive quality of energy. Oriental healers classified it under the tree energy category. The energy of barley is compatible to that of the liver and gallbladder. Hato mugi, or pearl barley, a species of wild barley originally grown in China, is especially charged with upward energy. Both regular and pearl barley can be eaten several times per week—in soup or cooked with other whole grains—in order to heal and nourish the liver and gallbladder. Barley tea, which is available in many natural food stores, also nourishes the liver and gallbladder and can be used as a daily beverage

Heart and Small Intestine Compared to the liver and gallbladder, the heart and small intestine have a more dynamic, active quality of energy. The heart is located in a yin position higher in the body, and is situated at the heart chakra, one of seven highly charged energy centers in the body. The heart and small intestine form a complementary unit. The heart is solid and compact (yang). Its main function is to distribute blood to organs and cells. The small intestine is a hollow tube (yin) in which nutrients are continually absorbed into the bloodstream. At the center of the small intestine is a highly charged region known as the hara chakra, another of the primary energy centers in the body.

Oriental healers referred to the highly active energy characteristic of the heart and small intestine as *fire energy*. Among the grains and their close relatives, corn, which is yin, is classified in the fire energy category. It nourishes and energizes the functions of the heart and small intestine. It can be eaten on a regular basis in the form of corn on the cob or used in such traditional dishes as polenta, whole corn meal, or grits.

Spleen, Pancreas, and Stomach The spleen, pancreas, and stomach are positioned on the left side of the body and are charged by downward or contracting energy that Oriental philosopher-healers referred to as *soil energy*. The spleen and pancreas have a compact, yang structure and are complementary to the stomach, which is a yin, hollow sac. Millet, a compact grain with a hard outer shell, is a product of downward or contracting energy and can be eaten on a regular basis to energize and strengthen these organs. Millet can be cooked with brown rice or added to vegetables to make delicious soups.

Lungs and Large Intestine The large intestine is located in the lower body where downward energy is stronger, and although it is long hollow tube, it is compressed into a small space. The lungs are complementary to the large intestine and contain many air sacs and blood vessels within in their spongy tissues. The lungs have a yang, compact structure, the large intestine, a yin, hollow form. Both represent gathering or condensing energy. Oriental healers named this stage *metal energy*. Brown rice, especially short grain rice, has strong condensed energy and corresponds to contracted metal energy. It can be eaten on a daily basis to strengthen and vitalize these organs.

Kidneys and Bladder The kidneys lie in the middle of the body; with one on the right and the other on the left. They have a yang, compact structure. The energy that nourishes the kidneys is like water, floating between yin and yang, or upward and downward movement, although on the whole, downward energy is slightly predominant. Oriental healers referred to this stage as *water energy*. Beans, which are more yang or contracted than most vegetables, and more yin or expanded than most grains, are an example of floating water energy. They strengthen and nourish the kidneys, and their complementary organ, the bladder. Small beans such as azuki and black soybeans have more concentrated energy and are especially beneficial. Beans and bean products can be eaten as a regular part of the diet. They are an excellent source of high-quality vegetable protein.

These five stages of energy are part of a a continuous cycle. In Oriental medicine, this cycle is known as *Go-Gyo*, or the "five transformations." The cycle of day and night and the changing of the seasons are examples of these five stages of change. During the course of the day, planetary energy constantly cycles back and forth. In the morning planetary energy moves in an upward direction. Morning corresponds to the stage tree energy. Planetary energy continues in an expansive direction through the morning and peaks at noon, the time of day that corresponds to fire energy. Planetary energy then changes direction, moving downward during the afternoon, the time of day corresponding to soil energy. Downward movement continues through the afternoon, so that by evening, the earth's atmosphere reaches its most condensed or contracted state. Evening corresponds to the metal stage. At night, the earth's atmosphere floats between heaven and earth, downward and upward energy. Night is the time of water energy.

The seasons also change in accord with the five transformations. Spring is the time of upward, or tree energy; summer, the time of active fire energy; late summer, the season of balanced, soil energy; autumn, the time of condensed, metal energy; and winter the time of floating energy. The cycle of solar energy, the carbon and nitrogen cycles, and the hydrological cycle are also examples of the movement of energy according to the five transformations. All things move and change in accord with the five energies.

The five transformations can also guide us in selecting vegetables and other foods for healing, and can help us utilize appropriate variety in our cooking methods. Leafy greens are charged with upward expansive energy (tree and fire). Contracted greens, such as turnip, daikon, carrot, and radish tops, are examples of tree energy. Broad leafy greens, such as mustard and collard greens, are examples of fire energy, as are celery, summer squash, cucumber, and other summer vegetables. Round vegetables, such as squash, onions, and cabbage are strongly charged with soil energy. Roots such as carrots, burdock, and daikon have even stronger yang energy (metal), while sea vegetables represent floating or water energy.

In cooking, we change the quality of our foods, by making their energies yin or yang. Methods such as quick steaming, blanching (quick boiling), and sauteing accelerate upward (tree) and active (fire) energy, while slow boiling, such as that used in making grain, bean, and vegetable stews, condenses the energy in food and corresponds to the soil stage. Pressure cooking is strongly contracting and corresponds to metal energy, while soup corresponds to the stage of water energy. Our bodies are comprised of all five energies, and to maintain optimal health, we need variety and balance in our diet. We need a wide variety of grains, beans, vegetables and cooking methods in order to provide the body with an adequate mix of energies.

The different aspects of our planetary environment can be classified according to the five transformations. The patterns of energy that create, nourish, and sustain our inner environment also function in our external environment. Certain parts of the environment are yin; others are yang. Trees and other forms of vegetation grow on the surface of the earth. Although they have roots, their main direction of growth is upward. They are the product of earth's expanding force, while animals are created primarily by contracting energy. Trees and other forms of vegetation correspond to the stage of upward or tree energy. Vegetation is a source of oxygen, a primary component of the atmosphere. The gaseous atmosphere surrounding the earth is also yin and can be classified in the tree energy category. Solar and other forms of energy are the most active and diffuse parts of our environment. They correspond to the stage fire energy, which is the most active and energized stage of the cycle.

Energy	Environment	Organs
Upward (Tree)	Vegetation growing on the surface of the earth; the atmosphere	Liver/gall-bladder
Active (Fire)	Solar and other forms of energy	Heart/small intestine
Downward (Soil)	The soil on the surface of the earth	Spleen (pancreas)/ stomach
Condensed (Metal)	Deposited resources within the earth (e.g., minerals, coal, oil, etc.)	Lung/large intestine
Floating (Water)	Oceans, lakes, rivers, and other bodies of water	Kidney/bladder

On the other hand, the soil on the surface of the earth has a solid and compact form. It corresponds to the stage of downward or soil energy. Metals and other minerals that are deposited deep within the earth are even more condensed than the soil at the surface. They correspond to the stage of condensed, metal energy. Rivers, lakes, and other bodies of water are examples of floating or water energy.

Our environment on earth is an organic whole, as is the human body. Each part of the environment is related to the others, just as each organ is connected to all the others. When we alter one part of the environment, the effects spiral outward and influence the environment as a whole. All things in the web of life are connected. For example, the burning of wood and other forms of plant matter releases carbon dioxide and other substances that alter the balance of the atmosphere (tree and fire energy). Airborne pollutants eventually fall to earth, changing the quality of the soil (soil energy). Pollution of the soil affects the quality of rivers, lakes, and other bodies of water on the earth (water energy), and that in turn affects trees and other forms of vegetation (tree energy). When plants are burned as fuel or decompose naturally, the cycle repeats.

The condition of the environment is a reflection of our personal health, including the condition of the internal organs. Our internal condition influences the way we relate to and manage the different aspects of our environment. If our health is good, our relationship with the environment is harmonious and self-sustaining. When our condition becomes stagnated and unhealthy, we relate to the environment in a wasteful, inefficient, and disruptive manner. How we relate to the environment is a function of not only our physical health, but our mental and emotional condition as well. Our mental and emotional responses are rooted in the condition of the internal organs, and the health of the organs is in turn determined by what we eat.

The spleen, pancreas, and stomach are related to the earth. Their condition influences our relationship with the soil, including our agricultural and farming practices. When these organs are sound and healthy, we prefer more natural methods of farming that maintain healthy, organic soil. When these organs become unbalanced, we lose confidence in natural farming and turn to pesticides and other chemicals that deplete the soil. In a similar way, the kidneys and bladder influence our relationship with water. Water pollution and the inefficient use of water resources are signs of widespread imbalance in the kidneys and bladder. This relationship works both ways: foods grown in chemically-depleted soil weaken the spleen, pancreas, and stomach, and chemically-treated or polluted water has a harmful effect on the kidneys and bladder.

Deforestation, including destruction of tropical rain forests, is a sign of widespread disorder in the liver and gall-bladder; while the use of non-renewable, highly polluting energy sources, such as fossil fuels and nuclear power, is evidence that many people are suffering from imbalance in the heart and small intestine. Over-consumption of meat and other forms of animal food is the primary cause of this imbalance. More than 92 percent of the energy consumed in the United States is from non-renewable resources. Depletion of the earth's mineral resources is an indication that many people are experiencing chronic imbalance in the lungs and large intestine.

The solution to the environmental crisis lies in restoring each of the organs, and the body as a whole, to a balanced healthy condition. The grains, vegetables, and other foods that heal the organs also heal the mind and emotions, as well as our relationship with our planetary environment. A naturally balanced, macrobiotic way of eating incorporates the understanding of food energetics and offers a practical way for everyone to restore harmony between their internal and external ecology. The macrobiotic way of life is thus the foundation of a new planetary medicine that can help us heal ourselves and the earth.

Afterword
A New Planetary Consciousness

From the depths of my being
I thank the earth, wind, and water.
I thank the sun, moon, and stars.
I thank the grains in the fields and the trees in the
    forest.
Because of them I am here.
I am one with the earth.
I am one with nature.
I am one with all forms of life.
Through my daily thoughts and actions
I vow to preserve and keep them for future
    generations.

December, 1991

All things are connected. Our thoughts and actions, no matter how small, affect everyone and everything.

We are all part of a vast spiral of life. Food, including air, water, and sunlight, is our link to the external world. Our daily foods are a product of nature, especially the world of vegetables. Plants are a product of the soil, water, and air, and these are made up of elements. The world of nature is made up of atoms, and these are composed of electrons, protons, and other vibrating particles. Underlying the material world is the world of energy or vibration. All things are part of this vibrating world. Waves of energy or vibration are the invisible threads that weave everything together in the fabric of existence. All vibrations are different appearances of two fundamental forces: expansion and contraction, beginning and end, short- and long-wave, yin and yang. These primary energies produce the endless cycles of expansion and contraction found everywhere, from the movement of carbon to the ebb and flow of the tides, from the rotation of the earth to the rhythm of the heart. Yin and yang arise continually from the infinite universe itself.

We cannot separate ourselves from the environment. Our environment on earth is the source of our life. Each world within the spiral of life is connected to all the others. The different realms of our environment are constantly in motion and continually change back and forth into one another. We are, in a sense, transformations of the environment. How we relate to the environment, therefore, is a reflection of how we relate to ourselves.

The quality of our environment determines the quality of our existence. If our environment is clean and pure, we can easily maintain health and happiness. If we spoil our environment, we easily become sick. Conversely, the quality of our environment is a reflection of our physical and mental condition. If we are healthy, so is our environment. If we become sick, either in body or mind, our environment begins to suffer.

Our life on this planet is brief in comparison to our endless spiritual journey. Human life is temporary in comparison to the life of planet earth. The succession of generations is based on a sacred trust. Each generation must care for and preserve the environment. It must not disrupt the balance of nature nor undercut the basis of life for future generations.

The environmental crisis is a product of shortsightedness over the past several centuries. The diet and way of life that gave rise to the modern crisis are a product of a view of life based on separateness rather than unity; a view of life based on unrealistic notions of self-importance and power.

Everything in this universe has a front and a back; a positive and negative side. The environmental crisis is the downside to the modern preoccupation with material prosperity, comfort, and convenience. Yet, the challenges ahead present us with unprecedented opportunities for growth and development. The environmental crisis is challenging us to reassess our modern view of life, and develop an awareness of nature and our place within it. At the same time, it is forcing us to examine the patterns of consumption that underlie modern life, and to change them to benefit ourselves and the earth. And, since it affects everyone on the earth, the environmental crisis challenges us to unite as one humanity in order to preserve our planetary home for generations yet unborn.

Appendix
Seven Precepts for Healing the Earth

1. We all share and are nourished by one planet, the earth.

2. By changing our diet and lifestyle, we have the power to change the environmental crisis into an opportunity for planetary healing and renewal.

3. The environmental crisis challenges all people to put aside their differences and unite to save the earth.

4. The environmental crisis offers a unique opportunity to establish health and peace on a planetary scale.

5. The environmental crisis is the downside to the modern pursuit of material prosperity, comfort, and convenience, including the modern diet.

6. The greater the threat of environmental destruction, the greater the need for personal reflection and change.

7. Environment destruction is now reaching a limit; a planetary revolution in consciousness, guided by the desire to live in harmony with the earth, is about to begin.

*Derived from the Seven Universal Principles of the Infinite Universe described by Michio Kushi in *The Book of Macrobiotics.*

Resources

One Peaceful World is an international information network and friendship society devoted to the realization of one healthy, peaceful world. Activities include educational and spiritual tours, assemblies and forums, international food aid and development, and publishing. Membership is $30/year for individuals and $50 for families and includes a subscription to the One Peaceful World Newsletter and a free book from One Peaceful World Press. For further information, contact:

> One Peaceful World
> Box 10, Becket, MA 01223
> (413) 623–2322
> Fax (413) 623–8827

The Kushi Institute offers ongoing classes and seminars, including cooking classes and workshops. For information, contact:

> Kushi Institute
> Box 7, Becket MA 01223
> (413) 623–5741
> Fax (413) 623–8827

Recommended Reading

1. Carson, Rachel. *Silent Spring* (Houghton-Mifflin, 1962).

2. Esko, Edward. *Basics and Benefits of Macrobiotics* (One Peaceful World Press, 1995).

3. Esko, Edward. *Healing Planet Earth* (One Peaceful World Press, first edition, 1992).

4. Esko, Edward. *Notes from the Boundless Frontier* (One Peaceful World Press, 1992).

5. Esko, Edward. *The Pulse of Life* (One Peaceful World Press, 1994).

6. Esko, Wendy. *Rice Is Nice* (One Peaceful World Press, 1995).

7. Esko, Wendy. *Soup du Jour* (One Peaceful World Press, 1996).

8. Gore, Al. *Earth in the Balance* (Plume, 1992).

9. Jack, Alex. *Inspector Ginkgo, The Macrobiotic Detective* (One Peaceful World Press, 1994).

10. Jack, Alex. *Let Food Be Thy Medicine* (One Peaceful World Press, 1994).

11. Jack, Alex. *Out of Thin Air: A Satire on Owls and Ozone, Beef and Biodiversity, Grains and Global Warming* (One Peaceful World Press, 1993).

12. Jack, Gale and Alex. *Amber Waves of Grain: American Macrobiotic Cooking* (Japan Publications, 1992).

13. Kushi, Aveline. *Aveline Kushi's Complete Guide to Macrobiotic Cooking* (with Alex Jack, Warner Books, 1985).

14. Kushi, Michio. *AIDS and Beyond* (with Alex Jack, One Peaceful World Press, 1995).

15. Kushi, Michio. *Basic Home Remedies* (One Peaceful World, 1994).

16. Kushi, Michio. *The Book of Macrobiotics* (with Alex Jack, Japan Publications, revised edition, 1986).

17. Kushi, Michio. *The Cancer-Prevention Diet* (with Alex Jack,

St. Martin's Press, 1983; revised and updated edition, 1993).

18. Kushi, Michio. *Diet for a Strong Heart* (with Alex Jack, St. Martin's Press, 1985).

19. Kushi, Michio. *Forgotten Worlds* (with Edward Esko, One Peaceful World Press, 1992).

20. Kushi, Michio. *The Gospel of Peace: Jesus's Teachings of Eternal Truth* (with Alex Jack, Japan Publications, 1992).

21. Kushi, Michio. *Healing Harvest* (with Edward Esko, One Peaceful World Press, 1994).

22. Kushi, Michio. *Holistic Health Through Macrobiotics* (with Edward Esko, Japan Publications, 1993).

23. Kushi, Michio. *Nine Star Ki* (with Edward Esko, One Peaceful World Press, 1991).

24. Kushi, Michio. *One Peaceful World* (with Alex Jack, St. Martin's Press, 1986).

25. Kushi, Michio. *The Philosopher's Stone* (with Edward Esko, One Peaceful World Press, 1994).

26. Kushi, Michio. *Spiritual Journey* (with Edward Esko, One Peaceful World Press, 1994).

27. King, F. H., *Farmers of Forty Centuries* (Rodale Press), original edition 1911.

28. Ohsawa, George. *Essential Ohsawa* (Avery Publishing Group, 1994).

29. Robbins, John. *Diet for a New America* (Stillpoint, 1987).

About the Author

Edward Esko began macrobiotic studies with Michio Kushi in 1971 and for twenty years has taught macrobiotic philosophy throughout the United States and Canada, as well as in Western and Eastern Europe, South America, Asia and the Far East. He has lectured on modern health issues and ecology at the United Nations in New York and is on the faculty of the Kushi Institute in Becket, Mass. He is the author of *Notes from the Boundless Frontier, The Pulse of Life,* and *Basics and Benefits of Macrobiotics,* and has co-authored or edited several popular books with Michio Kushi including *Holistic Health Through Macrobiotics.* He lives with his wife, Wendy, and their eight children in the Berkshires.

Index